RETAINING PROFESSIONAL NURSES
a planned process

RETAINING PROFESSIONAL NURSES
a planned process

JUDITH F. VOGT, Ph.D.

Associate Professor of Management,
College of Business, Department of Management,
The University of West Florida,
Pensacola, Florida

JOHN L. COX, Ph.D.

Associate Professor of Management,
College of Business, Department of Management,
The University of West Florida,
Pensacola, Florida

BETTY A. VELTHOUSE, R.N., M.S.N.

Visiting Professor, College of Business,
Department of Management,
The University of West Florida,
Pensacola, Florida

BARBARA H. THAMES, R.N., M.B.A.

Assistant Director of Nursing,
West Florida Hospital,
Pensacola, Florida

with **31** illustrations

The C. V. Mosby Company

ST. LOUIS • TORONTO • LONDON   1983

MOSBY

A TRADITION OF PUBLISHING EXCELLENCE

Editor: Michael R. Riley
Assistant editor: Sally Gaines
Manuscript editor: Judy Jamison
Design: Jeanne Bush
Production: Kathleen L. Teal, Teresa Breckwoldt, Judy Bamert

The C.V. Mosby Company
11830 Westline Industrial Drive, St. Louis, Missouri 63141

Library of Congress Cataloging in Publication Data

Main entry under title:

Retaining professional nurses.

  Bibliography: p.
  Includes index.
  1. Nurses—Employment. 2. Health facilities
—Personnel management. 3. Labor turnover.
I. Vogt, Judith F. [DNLM: 1. Nursing—Organiza-
tion. 2. Personnel management. WY 30 R437]
RT86.7.R46 1983 362.1′73′0683 82-14159
ISBN 0-8016-5226-X

VT/VH/VH 9 8 7 6 5 4 3 2 1 01/A/054

To those professionals who have touched our lives
and made this endeavor meaningful and cogent
and who have given us the impetus for completion.

Delores, Larry, Madeline, Judy,
Vicky, Ken, Diane, Ruth, Kay, Usha,
Virginia, Marilyn, Sherry, Phyllis, Cynthia,
Beth, Peter, Paulette, Mary, Madelyn, Kathy, Pat,
Carmen, Jack, John, Jo, Linda, Joe, Barry, Joani, Romona,
Sandy, Annie Mac, Mary Jo, Justo, Nita, Edna, Charlotte, Sally, Fran,
Carol, Connie, Vickie, Jean, Sharon, Janis, Janet, Faye, Sharon, Norma, Karen

PREFACE

This book goes beyond simplistic and narrow solutions to solve the problems of nursing shortage and turnover. Our book, in fact, demonstrates that there is no shortage of nurses; however, their turnover and dropout rates are high. We explore and document the reasons for and consequences of these problems from financial, managerial, organizational, and professional viewpoints.

It is our perspective that retention strategies that work are those that are (1) planned according to the needs and circumstances of the specific facility, (2) constantly assessed and updated, and (3) based upon such principles of human resource management as staff development, team building and enhanced communications, and skilled, growing, effective managers. We also imply, through the use of the positive word "retention," that only healthy components—guidelines and activities—are appropriate to the objective. We are proactive (to retain) versus reactive (to recruit or to cope with turnover). We focus on opportunities and innovations and the roles of hospital administration and nursing administration as well as those of the head nurse and supervisor.

Our purpose in writing this book is to provide those individuals concerned with the retention of nurses more creative and innovative approaches to keeping nurses in the profession and work force. Our biases stem from our education, experiences, and belief systems. An educator, an industrial engineer, a management consultant, and a nurse manager bring their insights and orientations to the issues and practical resolutions of high turnover. Our common thread, which we transmit through this book, is the belief that professional people want to grow, want to contribute, and want to be valued, and that health care organizations that foster and encourage these human conditions will retain productive, self-fulfilled nurse professionals.

A major strength of this book lies in our broad backgrounds. We offer a unique blend of theoretician/practitioner/educator with industrial, organizational, and academic experience. The result is a book that combines the philosophical aspects of people management with practical and proved methods for increasing nurse retention. A second strength of the book is its emphasis on contemporary, innovative, and utilitarian approaches and strategies for increased retention. Third, our book offers a conceptual framework as well as specific suggestions. This allows its readership the opportunity to explore other alternatives within a theoretical structure. Additional contributions to theory will be generated by others as they define their position. Fourth, the book offers recommendations directly applicable to both the process and content of retention program design. It speaks to issues related to developing a tailor-made approach for the best fit in each organization while it offers specific activities and insights relevant to first-line supervisors, middle managers, chief administrators, and boards of directors.

This book began with four professionals who had an idea. We came together, nurturing the idea and our own unique perspectives derived from our own backgrounds, education, and experiences. Throughout the writing we have valued each other's opinions, ideas, disagreements, work schedules, feedback, work styles, and end-points. We have valued our differences and recognized the core of our similarities. We each have grown and we each have learned. The outcome is a major contribution to health care which was supported by attending to process issues of our relationships. We believe our efforts to be of the highest quality.

We appreciate our colleagues at The University of West Florida for creating a climate conducive to the pursuit of achievement. Members of the Management Department, especially Ralph Roberts, Chairman, as well as Richard Einbecker, Dean of the College of Business, and Dr. Arthur Doerr, Vice President for Academic Affairs, have been particularly supportive of this endeavor. In addition, West Florida Hospital and its administration and staff have been important to our efforts and deserves special attention. We thank them all.

We also want to recognize our publisher, The C.V. Mosby Company, for its valuing and support of this project as well as for its outstanding attention to its responsibilities. Of most significance to us were Chester Dow, Senior Editor, Nursing Sciences Division, and Sally Gaines, Assistant to the Senior Editor. Chet has been exceptional from our first interaction with him—his professional demeanor corresponded with our hopes for the book.

Several persons have typed or administered the details of the project; they include Z (Zenobia) Milhouse, Ileana Martinez, Marie Glass, Cindy Watford, and Debra Hyder. They were committed to a professional representation of our efforts and have so performed.

And for each of us there have been significant, supportive, and special people:

For Judy, her co-authors—Betty, Barbara, and Lew—and Professor Allen Menlo of the University of Michigan, her mentor.

For Betty, her sister, Chuckie, who always asks, "How is your writing?"

For Barbara, Virginia Williams, Director of Nursing, Jack Bovender, Administrator, and Cynthia Ayres, for her creative input in figure designs—all from West Florida Hospital.

For John L. (Lew), Linda and Jeff for their patience.

Judith F. Vogt
John L. Cox
Betty A. Velthouse
Barbara H. Thames

CONTENTS

RETAINING
PROFESSIONAL NURSES
a planned process

1

OVERVIEW

INTRODUCTION: OUR PERSPECTIVE AND PHILOSOPHY
NURSING: A HISTORICAL PERSPECTIVE
DESCRIPTION OF THE PROBLEM
    Impact of a myriad of forces
    The women's movement
    Crisis management orientation
    Causes and roots of turnover
THE IMPACT OF TURNOVER
    Financial
    Productivity
    Staff maturity
    Growth (turnover as a positive force) and non growth
    Disillusionment
    Prestige of the profession
A CONCEPTUAL CONCLUSION
    Efficiency and effectiveness defined
    . . . And the retention of nurses

INTRODUCTION: OUR PERSPECTIVE AND PHILOSOPHY

Nurses are plentiful. Enough qualified, educated practitioners exist to provide excellent patient care to all hospital (institutionalized) patients. In the early 1950s, it was reported that there were more nurses who did not practice their profession than those who did.[14] This trend has not diminished; a study in 1976 estimated that 55% of all qualified nurses did not practice nursing.[2] This behavior is compounded by (and probably interrelated with) nursing's struggle for identity in the health care industry as well as by the increased variety of professional opportunities recently opened to women. The "nursing shortage" has reached crisis proportions. Yet, it does not exist.

In 1973 it was estimated that 68 to 75% of all employed nurses worked in hospital (institutional) settings.[12] This environment epitomizes the essence and experience of nursing care to many nurses. There are many nurses who find this the most rewarding arena in which to practice, many who find the structure and security of the hospital optimum for their work. The nurses practicing in this setting, however, experience frustration, disillusionment, and value conflict. Hospital surveys report turnover of up to 50% annually (in 1955, 67%; in 1962, 58%; in 1965, 58%; in 1970, in multiple surveys, 40%, 100%, 70%; in 1974, 35 to 60% and 15 to 57%). To provide these nurses with fulfillment, job satisfaction, reward and value, growth options, respect, and a desire to continue in nursing, is the emphasis of this book.

The answer to the nursing shortage does not lie in increased numbers, or in innovative nurse preparation schemes, or in grander recruitment practices. Since the early 1960s the number and variety of nurse preparation programs have grown explosively. Controversy, antagonism, and rivalry continue between the diploma graduate, the baccalaureate graduate, the 27-month RN, and the 5-year program graduate. The role of and need for the LPN and the nurse's assistant are discussed repeatedly and at high levels. Although these issues need resolution, they are beyond the scope of this manuscript because we believe they do not significantly affect nurse attrition and turnover. Emphasis will be put on the quality of the individual nurse's contribution and the reward attached to that contribution, rather than the quantity of nurses that can be generated.

Monies are being spent lavishly on recruitment. Advertisements are large, offering such enticements as bonuses, bounties, lengthy orientations, and internships. Much of this effort, time, and money is wasted because recruitment does not have a partner in retention. There is little thought of, plan for, or work toward retention. Recruitment and retention must be congruent. The hiring of personnel "implies a social obligation on the part of the organization to take reasonable steps to ensure the continuity of employment as well as an economic obligation."[21] Few hospitals are oriented toward fulfilling this social obligation. A high degree of retention is not accidental. It does not coexist with an attitude of acceptance; that is, "our turnover rate is only 30%, which is within the national average, so we do not have a problem." Turnover represents a failure on the part of the organization in selection, placement, orientation, supervision, or challenge.

Turnover is costly, and it is contagious. It is imperative therefore that turnover be thoroughly investigated. Preestablished criteria must be outlined for both acceptable and unacceptable turnover. Each nurse has an individual reason or combination of reasons for leaving a job. It is therefore important that each case of turnover be analyzed. When statistics on turnover are collected, voluntary and involuntary turnover must be separated. Karl D. Bays, in his address to the National Conference on Nursing in 1981, stated that the nursing shortage in this country will not be solved until we learn to ask the "right questions. One important question is whether we have often enough asked nurses themselves about their roles, their motivations, their goals and ideas."[3] Turnover is also necessary for the health and well-being of the organization. "As less qualified people leave, openings are created for more qualified replacements. If the process functions well, the organization is continually revitalized and upgraded."[20] A complacent attitude toward turnover suggests and leads to a diminished value of and investment in the employee (the nurse), which contributes to the problem. Further, it puts the organization in a dependent, passive, and reactive position at a time when health care desperately needs a proactive and independent posture.

High turnover has become an accepted fact in health care. It is accepted because 98% of nurses are women and because it is a profession that has been historically dependent on the physician. But the most significant reason turnover remains an accepted fact of health care is that to attack the problem would involve planning, commitment, cooperation, and change within an entire organization. Nurse shortage and nursing turnover have been recognized as a critical combination. It became crucial primarily when the turnover-shortage phenomenon began causing the closure of hospital units and putting a strain on the hospital budget by consuming large amounts of money for supplementary agency nurses. Turnover is a serious, alarming problem.

Some of the known causes of nurse turnover include frustration, boredom, apathy, value conflict, rotation of shifts, powerlessness, lack of recognition, "burnout," unrelenting stress, low salaries, conflict between professional excellence and promotion criteria, poor definition and role clarity within professional hierarchy, and conflict between physicians and nurses. The complexity, diversity, and importance of the issues involved dictate an in-depth, long-range approach to solution and resolution. The strategy must be focused on both individuals and the organization, must include both short-term and long-range project perspectives, and must contain elements of ongoing individual, departmental, and organizational assessment. A concerted effort to fix nursing turnover necessarily involves change, conflict, growth, commitment, consistency, creativity, ambiguity, flexibility, and productivity. It is not an undertaking to be assumed lightly or a decision for one person alone to make. It goes beyond monthly in-service education and orientation; it involves attitudes, beliefs, personal needs, patterns, values, territoriality, milieu, and organization dynamics. It involves participants/ employees in multidisciplinary proactive planning, discussion, and change. Effective strategies will create stress within individuals, departments, and the organization. There is a need to build in mechanisms and forums for dealing with the anxiety, ambiguity, and ambivalence prompted by corrective efforts.

Nursing turnover–nurse shortage is a threat to our present system of health care delivery. Some type of change is necessary. Professional nurse continuity enriches the organization in community regard, in professional reputation, in consumer evaluations, and in increased revenue. The benefits of increased efficiency, profitability, productivity, morale, and growth provided by a stable work force have been demonstrated repeatedly by industry.[18] The stable professional staff is even more significant.

Retention is planned. It is obvious in an organization's mission statement and in an administrator's philosophy, as well as in the organization's policies and procedures, supervisory job descriptions, performance appraisal mechanisms, conflict resolution tactics, and its methods for self-evaluation. This book will address itself to *planned retention*. Chapter 1 explores the history of, present state of, and impact of the problem. Chapter 2 identifies entry components in the "life cycle" of the employee consistent with planned retention. Chapter 3 explores the various roles in the supervisory process and their impact on retention. Chapter 4 is devoted to motivation. Chapter 5 considers strategies for individual development. Chapter 6 recognizes the environmental and multidisciplinary aspects of health care and their responsibilities to and interdependence with retention. Chapter 7 reports innovations and possibilities. Chapter 8 examines the theory and process of applied change; it also defines requisite skills for those who choose the role of change agent in terms of planned retention within the profession, the practice, and the organizational life of nursing.

From 1950 to the present, the literature and research have demonstrated the importance of planning, of shared problem solving, of commitment to the personal needs of employees, and of collaboration among groups. We have been made aware of the value of asking the questions: Where are we? Where do we want to be? It is the *process* of asking and answering these questions by organizations that will promote the resolution of the problem of retention while increasing and advocating the *quality* of work and work life within nursing. Our book speaks to these concepts and this process.

NURSING: A HISTORICAL PERSPECTIVE

To understand more fully the circumstances in which professional nursing finds itself today vis-à-vis retention, and to appreciate the evolution of nursing as a predominately female profession (thus further impacting on retention), it is necessary to explore the past. Before proceeding, however, a distinction must be drawn between nursing and *professional* nursing. Nursing, in the sense of caring for the sick, has its roots in antiquity; nursing activities provided one of the natural advantages of belonging to early social structures. As individuals within social groups demonstrated an adeptness for caring for the sick, they would be called on to nurse friends, family, and acquaintances; through this tending behavior they established the reputation and the "practice" of nursing.

When viewed historically, the development of nursing and women's integral relationship with it seems to fall into three periods: (1) from the earliest times until the latter part of the eighteenth century (around 1775); (2) from the latter part of the eighteenth century until the first modern school for nurses at St. Thomas Hospital, England, in 1860; and (3) from 1860 until the present.[15] The first suggestion of women being associated with the healing arts is found in Greek mythology. Asklepios, the first physician (who was eventually deified), had six daughters of whom one, Hygeia, became goddess of health; another daughter became the restorer of health, and yet another the preserver of health.[15] Until the Christian era, there is little evidence to support the existence of any organized group of nurses, male or female. With the advent of the Christian era, however, there began a new spirit. As the church preached the ideals of brotherhood and service, charity and self-sacrifice, groups of workers were formed whose main function was to care for the sick and needy. As an offshoot of this activity, nursing of the poor became a popular way of atoning for sin. Nursing was regarded as a paramount duty of the church, and with the rise of monasticism the care of the sick became the function of many religious orders of men and women. Nursing care provided by Catholic orders progressed, but in countries where Catholic organizations were upset by the Reformation, nursing sank to its lowest levels. This was especially true in England. The new Protestant Church had no use for cloisters and religious institutions, and felt no responsibility to the sick as had the early Catholic Church.

A significant factor in nursing's evolution was the status of women in the social structure of two or three centuries ago. From the antiquity of Rome to the Middle Ages, the Catholic Church had assigned a place in society to women that afforded them much freedom and opportunity; and lay nursing orders also allowed women to contribute. The Protestant Church, although it stood for freedom of thought and freedom of religion, did not think much of freedom for women. A career in nursing would have been unthinkable for a respectable woman in the year 1700.

During the nineteenth century, nurses increased their practical experience in caring for the sick, although there was still no concept of scientific medicine, of personal or social standing, or of responsibility. They were primarily limited to duties such as attending to the physical needs of the patient and seeing that the patient was reasonably clean, although even this was not considered essential. Thus the concept of the *art* of nursing (based on technique, craft) had its beginning, but the *science* of nursing had yet to evolve. But as medicine and surgery advanced, so did nursing. In fact advances such as improved sanitation, nutrition, and hospital facilities began to aid the development of nursing. Professional nursing has been and probably always will be closely allied with medical progress and practice.

Some 160 years ago the Industrial Revolution was in full swing in Europe and the United States, but hospitals of that period were wretched dumping places for the poor. Sanitation was unknown; patients were rarely bathed, linen seldom changed, and surgery (primarily limited to amputations) combined risk with torture. Often the disease that brought the patients to the hospital was not what killed them; instead it was infection. In hospitals of that day, the care was administered by women who were paupers, drunkards, or prostitutes—basically those who were unfit for other work. This work was often punishment for the women and, as a result, they victimized rather than cared for their charges. For example, it was not unheard of for the nurse to rob or physically abuse the patient. It seems that under these deplorable conditions only a major revolution could change the situation. That such a revolution took place and the third period in the history of nursing was initiated is now known. That it was brought about through the efforts of an English gentlewoman is, however, little short of a miracle.[9]

The concept of nursing as an economic, independent, and secular vocation, an art requiring intelligence and technical skill as well as devotion and moral purpose, was first developed by Florence Nightingale. One of the major problems that Florence had to deal with in pursuing her vocation was that of combating the objections of family members. Florence Nightingale, born in 1820, overcame her parent's objections and society's valuation of nursing and prepared herself for what she considered her vocation and God's calling: to improve the quality of hospitals and of nursing care. Her family's opposition persisted, causing her much frustration and probably accounting for the various psychosomatic ailments she suffered throughout her life. At age 31 Florence Nightingale went to Kaiserwerth, Germany, to work and study under Pastor Fliedner. It was during this period that she found compassionate attitudes sorely lacking in the hospitals she visited. Also at this point she began to realize the importance of systematic nursing based on knowledge of (1)

the body and (2) disease processes and how to treat them. It was this awareness that now clarified her mission and identified what was missing from nursing of that day. Soon after leaving Kaiserwerth in 1853, she persuaded her
father to give her a yearly allowance when she was offered the position in
London of superintendent of the Institution for Sick Gentlewomen in Dis-
tressed Circumstances. This job paid no salary; she even had to pay the salary
of her personal housekeeper, who came along to keep her "respectable." In
this, her first real job, she proved to be an expert at administration and innovation. Dramatic changes were made in sanitation, nutrition, and attitude.
She initiated rounds among the patients and expressed care, concern, and
empathy. Additionally, she continued the habit of observing and taking notes
that she had begun in Kaiserwerth. Although Miss Nightingale made significant progress in England during this time, a historical event far from England
had a more significant effect on the course of nursing's history: the Crimean
War. With her contingent of nurses, she instituted innovations and made significant contributions to the care of the wounded soldiers during the Crimean
conflict. As a result of her work, far-reaching reforms were undertaken. Female army nursing was firmly established. Nutrition was improved with the
introduction of special diet kitchens, and a measure of cleanliness was provided by the nurses. Construction and regulations were changed and
improved in both barracks and hospitals, and provisions were made for rec-
reation and entertainment of the soldiers when off duty. An army medical
school was established and special instructions given to selected soldiers who
became the first corpsmen trained to give skilled care to the sick and
wounded.[9]

During these years the long hours, the fear of failure, and her mother and
sister's nonsupportive, inconsiderate behavior combined to adversely affect
Florence Nightingale's health. But still she persevered. Her reputation grew
and she was called on to consult in many areas. It also became clear to her that
if nursing was to progress as she envisioned it, there must be a systematic way
of training qualified nurses. The first experiment in formal nursing education
was undertaken at St. Thomas Hospital, London. With the public monies that
had been given to Miss Nightingale in honor of her contribution to the war,
the school was launched. The school was an immediate success, and the graduates, called "Nightingales," were sought after in Australia, France, and the
United States. They were especially in demand to assist in setting up schools
based on the Nightingale plan.

Florence Nightingale lived to see nursing develop to the point that its
leaders were looking toward professional organization and official recognition of the profession through governmental licensure. An interesting side-
light is that she was opposed to licensure on the basis that the art of nursing
could not be demonstrated through a standardized exam. Licensure, how-

ever, became a reality in England 9 years after her death. More than a century ago Florence Nightingale expounded the philosophy of flexibility that still guides nursing today: "Everything which succeeds is not the production of scheme (plan), or rules or regulations made beforehand, but a mind observing and adapting itself to wants and events."[9] Her legacy to nursing—of knowledge, humanitarianism, and compassion—is timeless.

With all of the reforms and advancements of nursing and medicine evidenced in hospital settings during the late nineteenth and early twentieth centuries, it was only natural that progress would not remain within the confines of the hospital and sickroom. Medicine and nursing developed, and their purpose spread beyond the cure of disease; they began to be concerned with its very prevention. To prevent disease required that attention be paid to the healthy in the communities, schools, and army camps. Laboratories that aided in the control of disease did not have to be housed in hospitals. And as more and more attention was given to keeping people well, the new science of public health was born. The relatively simple measures devised by physicians to protect the population as a whole could just as well be administered by trained assistants, and nurses became the logical group to assume this role. Thus the public health nurse came to be. Nursing was expanding its function and growing rapidly in size and responsibilities.

The Red Cross, inspired by Florence Nightingale, had its origin in Italy in 1859. As an international institution it was invaluable in times of war, but it also assumed many peacetime activities. It was entirely independent and supported by voluntary contributions. In 1881 Clara Barton founded the American Red Cross. The formation of the American Nurses' Association in 1911 marked the beginning of the world's now largest professional women's organization and established the nursing profession as a social entity. At the same time, state nurses' associations promoted state laws to regulate nursing practice.[6] The need to protect the public from incompetent practitioners was recognized by the profession as one of their responsibilities, and this was a way to assure it.

The next major historical events that impacted on nursing were World Wars I and II. World War I created an immense demand for nurses, made new fields of specialization available, and created a public awareness of the importance of effective nursing. The first World War affected Britain more profoundly than the United States. Nursing resources were drained to a point below the minimum requirements of civilian hospitals. Following the war, British nursing continued to suffer from a lack of recruits, which was a vital defect. The development of Canadian nursing closely paralleled that in the United States, whereas nursing's beginnings in other areas of the world were largely pioneered by missionary nurses from England and the United States. World War II had a still more far-reaching impact on nursing. Directly or indirectly, World War II affected nearly every dimension of the lives of the U.S. citizens. Nowhere were the demands or changes more drastic than in the areas of nursing and medicine. In combat, RNs were forced to accept many duties and responsibilities relegated to them that previously they had been forbidden to carry out or were thought incapable of doing. It was at this time that the shortage of RNs at home prompted the introduction of semiprofessionals (e.g., nurse aides, licensed vocational nurses, technicians), a change that was not retracted at war's end. Of the significant changes in nursing resulting from World War II, one of the most meaningful was that government for the first time recognized RNs as a group and concerned itself with their advancement.

The postwar era of new medicines, new techniques, and new equipment brought a new awareness into hospitals, and nurses along with other health professionals found it impossible to resume prewar ways of nursing.

Beginning in the late nineteenth century, changes in the nursing profession had been reflected in the changing patterns of nursing education. By the time of the Civil War, the American Medical Association's Committee for the Training of Nurses recommended that schools of nursing be established in connection with hospitals. Three schools were established in 1873 based on Miss Nightingale's principles. Because of a lack of private funds for their support, they were absorbed by the hospitals with which they affiliated. Although there was dissatisfaction with this arrangement, this type of school continued to proliferate. Goldmark[11] criticized this pattern of nursing preparation because it defined nursing on an apprenticeship basis, a method long since abandoned by other professions that required specialized education.

A study by social anthropologist Esther Brown in 1948 expanded awareness of the inadequacies in nursing when she found prewar hospital training programs inadequate for professional nurses who were destined to be the planners and supervisors of patient care.[4] She recommended that nursing be included within college curriculums to combat the lack of awareness within nursing of the broader developments and advances in health care and of far-reaching, rapidly changing social issues. Brown's findings were paralleled in another study by an economist who corroborated the fact that most RNs lacked the educational background of other professional groups and that nursing was facing great problems (e.g., identity as a profession, fragmentation of the practitioners). In 1965 the American Nurses' Association (ANA) prepared a position paper that reiterated the position that nursing education should take place in institutions of higher learning within the general system of education. This perspective was accepted by the ANA membership in 1966, although far from unanimously. The primary purpose (and outcomes) of that ANA position paper was to force public education to assume responsibility for the education of the nursing professionals and to assure students in nursing that their programs could be equated academically with those of other professions. Three programs to prepare nurses have been developed and are presently operative: the hospital diploma school, the associate degree (AD) program at junior colleges, and the bachelor of science in nursing (BSN) degree program at universities. All of these programs prepare nurses for entry level positions in nursing, and all graduates must take the same licensing examination. The present nurse preparation dilemma and the studies that have been done revolving around the entry level into practice are all logical, scientific, and reasonable, but they have not served to unify the profession. Rather, the varied approaches have done much to fragment and divide the nursing professionals. This phenomenon of ongoing fragmentation is a characteristic typical of developing groups. One of the issues of this fragmentation is career mobility. Career mobility continues to be difficult for the nurse without the generic baccalaureate degree in nursing. Nurses with other degrees (e.g., behavioral science, education, business) are often devalued or ignored by nursing leaders and educators. In studying the history of professional nursing one becomes aware that through the fight for professional advancement, the struggle for the political, economic, and educational freedom of women is entangled. In no other occupation or profession has the emancipation of women been of greater or more practical significance.[15]* Women have always held a very precarious position in the labor market. As have minorities, women have been expendable, to be used or rejected depending on fluctuations in the marketplace. Now employers in most areas of the country are aggressively seeking nurses. This does not imply, however, that discrimination is less or that changes are not needed. The implications are evident. Nurses today have more opportunity to initiate changes within the health care system than at any time since the early part of this century.[5] How they handle this challenge, united or divided, will greatly influence the future of professional nursing in the United States.

Although women often leave nursing (to devote 5 or 10 years to child rearing, for instance), most return eventually. There are more divorcees and single mothers in nursing than in any other profession. The nurse today is not the old-fashioned, traditional female of yesteryear, subservient to the health care system and working only for a second income. Nursing is now advancing into the area of independent practice with nurse clinicians, nurse practitioners, and clinical specialists. Opportunities exist for nurses to prepare themselves educationally among numerous specialty choices in a wide variety of settings.

*The impact of the women's movement on retention is explored later in this chapter. It is beyond the scope of this book, however, to trace the historical events in women's efforts toward economic and professional equality.

CURRENT NURSING ISSUES

Entry level into practice (AD, diploma, BSN)
Accreditation, licensure, certification
National credentialing center
Institutional licensure
Medical versus nursing control of advanced registered nurse practitioners
Nurse practice acts and enlightened legislators
Nursing diagnosis and nursing process—a basis for practice
Collegiality with physicians—shared decision-making responsibility
Professional leadership—training, experience, perspective

Although nurses face challenges from government, physicians, hospitals, and other agencies for the control of their practice, their greatest problem in advancing the profession is caused by the dissension and fragmentation within the ranks of the nursing population itself. A summary of the current issues facing nursing can be found above; it reemphasizes the most basic and sophisticated of choices to make and concerns to be explored facing this developing profession. In some instances the turmoil and dissension in nursing is encouraged and even perpetuated by hospital and nursing administrations through inflexibility in scheduling, vindictive discipline, unfair wage and salary administration, poor human relations, and lack of respect for each other as colleagues and peers. These behaviors plus others indicate a lack of professional management perspective, and this lack has greatly contributed to the high rates of turnover among professional nurses. It is the defining of nursing management's roles and responsibilities that nurses now face.

If nursing is to progress, then the implications from the past must be recognized and dealt with in a direct manner by all who have the power to influence nursing's future. This means that change, regardless of how painful, must take place not only in the work setting but in the minds and philosophies of those who practice the profession. Current directions for such change include these:

- All of nursing's diverse constituencies must consider joining together as a means of supporting and promoting common national policies dealing with licensure, practice standards, education, and credentialing.
- Nursing must explore the involvement and role of nursing administration as a part of top management teams in health care settings.
- Salaries, benefits, and educational opportunities for nurses must be reviewed and expanded in light of the responsibilities of nurses.

- Physicians and nurses must redefine their partnership, with nurses exploring their roles in clinical decision making in terms of authority and responsibility for their practice.

It is the attainment of unity and implementation of the above activities that remain the next formidable tasks for nursing. We believe our comments, perspectives, and suggestions related to retention can make a significant contribution to this effort, because we value nursing, its role, its membership, and its struggle toward self-worth.

DESCRIPTION OF THE PROBLEM

The "problem" addressed in this book is really made up of two sides of the same coin; the problems of nursing turnover and the attendant perceived shortage of nursing personnel. Together they represent a major challenge to hospital administrators.

Turnover of nursing personnel in this country, both at the first-line supervisory (head nurse) and at the individual contributor (professional staff nurse) level, is of major interest. Quoted turnover rates range from about 35 to 200%, depending on the hospital and its location. High turnover is a problem in *any* labor-intensive industry, and health care is definitely labor intensive. A recent report indicates that about 50% of a hospital's budget is for its payroll and that more than 70% of this figure is for nurses' salaries.

Figures for 1981 indicate there are approximately 1.4 million nurses currently employed in the profession. Although some sources quote turnover rates as high as 70% per year (Dr. Jerome Lysaught), let us assume a 50% rate for the sake of a numerical example. A 50% turnover rate of 1.4 million nurses employed means about 700,000 nurses change jobs each year. An often-quoted value for turnover cost is $2500 per nurse. Multiplying this figure by the turnover number gives a dollar value of $1.75 billion for nursing turnover per year—a staggering cost.

Every nurse who leaves a job creates an opening that must be filled. Attempting to fill the position brings the hospital face to face with the other facet of the same problem, the nursing shortage. This shortage situation has existed for a number of years but has gained national prominence over the past several years. Taken by itself, the nursing shortage is certainly not unique. In the past few decades cycling shortages have developed in various types of personnel. For instance, there have been at least three periods since 1960 when someone with an engineering degree was "hot." Much the same is true of teachers below the university level; there were too few, then far too many. The one professional personnel area where the shortage of practitioners appears to be perennial is in nursing. What makes the nursing shortage unique is the fact that it does not exist. On the one hand, we have an official of the ANA reported as testifying before Congress to a shortage of 40,000 to 60,000 nurses. On the other hand, we have a nursing official in a metropolitan area quoted as saying that if every nurse in the area worked only 1 day per week, there would be no nursing shortage in the city.

This apparent contradiction, coupled with the continued strain on the health care facility to maintain an adequate staff of nurses, has led to the national attention focused on the problem.

Impact of a myriad of forces

Most of the causes of the *apparent* nursing shortage are interrelated. These include, but are not limited to the following.

The declining Florence Nightingale effect. In the beginning of the profession (and indeed, until the last 20 years or so), nurses were thought to be born for the profession and were expected to be willing to work for low pay. Dedicated to the care of their patients, nurses were thought to be uninterested in money or in the other material and mundane things in life.

As a result of various changes in our society, people in general are no longer expected to take a vow of poverty to work in their chosen professions. Add to this the number of nurses who are sole supporters of a family and cannot afford to work for inadequate remuneration, and there is a double reason for people to leave relatively low-paying professions like nursing.

Other doors have opened. Women, who primarily comprise the profession of nursing, are now accepted in many other professions that have been closed to them in the past. They no longer must stick to traditional women's careers such as teaching and nursing. Indeed women cannot legally be restricted into or out of any profession, and actuality is not far behind.

Accountability. Accountability has become an issue in areas that have heretofore been almost sacred. As late as the 1940s no one really questioned the judgment or actions of a doctor or nurse. Now the frequency of lawsuits and the sizes of the judgments awarded amply demonstrate the end of the untouchable era.

Health care consumers are better educated concerning their rights as patients. Various media regularly carry health care information for the consumer; hospitals have put greater emphasis on patient education (such as the Patient's Bill of Rights), and interest groups—professional, governmental, or otherwise—continue to press for greater accountability within the caring professions. These outside pressures, plus continued and heightened interest by the members to police their own profession, have combined to place nursing in almost a fishbowl atmosphere.

Responsibility without authority. Basic management textbooks state that to be put in a position of being responsible for something without having the authority to control it puts one in an *untenable* position. Nurses have much responsibility for patient care but, in general, have little decision-making authority.

It remains a unique event when even experienced, competent, and well-trained nurses are recognized as such by physicians. In addition, some organizational policies and procedures do not permit the breadth of judgment and decision-making allowed by nurses' education and knowledge. A further complication is the (sometimes) lack of professional recognition accorded staff nurses within their own ranks by their peers and supervisors. These conditions often put the staff nurse and head nurse in an extremely frustrating position. Criticisms of them run from not taking enough action in one patient's behalf to taking too much action (latitude) on behalf of another.

Emotionalism. The joint problems of nursing turnover and shortages are amplified by the fact that health care in general is such an emotion-charged issue. Each of us wants health care (of whatever type we need) to be available to us, close to us, around the clock, 7 days a week. For virtually all other service industries, the problem of turnover and/or a personnel shortage does not have the same emotional impact. In a restaurant or retail sales situation, for instance, if service is slow and we are told that someone has called in sick or just did not show up, we wryly shake our heads and philosophize about how people just are not dependable and interested in their working life. In schools, colleges, and universities, when we are short-staffed, we allow larger classes and persevere. In health care we tend to take a personnel shortage a good deal more personally. Generally if we are at a hospital looking for service, we are there to get service for someone for whom we care a great deal (a friend, a relative, or ourselves). If the expected care is not immediately forthcoming, we tend to become indignant and loud.

As people we tend to support the nurses' rights to good working conditions at a fair salary. Yet, as consumers of health care, we immediately think negatively of any action that smacks of rising prices and lowered availability of care. Nurses, in turn, must think in terms of patient care, yet must also consider the necessity of earning a livable wage while working toward improving the conditions under which they work. Attempts to improve conditions (say through a union) may generate a great deal of negative publicity.

The women's movement

The women's movement has added to the impetus to write this book. The women's movement as discussed here is considered to be a conglomeration of historical issues and happenings, including the following:

- The realization and valuing of women, by themselves as well as others, as worthwhile and coequal individuals—the self-assessment and resulting conclusions of self-worth being experienced by women from all levels of society, leading to their expectation of coequal treatment in all facets of their work life

- The development of networking—the concept and process of relationship building, used so long in male-dominated work forces, broadening and supporting the growth of women and the women's movement itself
- As discussed previously, the movement of women into the position of being heads of households, plus the opening up to women of careers that had been closed to them
- The legal requirement that women be treated as equals with men in terms of salary and job opportunity—the increasing realization by women that they do have a legal and effective recourse when treated badly, plus a greater willingness to confront their derogators, greatly enhancing the forward movement of women

Nurses in a hospital setting have had difficulty in realizing the benefits of the women's movement because of traditions and hierarchies built up over time. Perhaps the chief contribution of this book will be the presentation of the methods by which a nurse or group of nurses can rise above their day-to-day conflicts and work toward a permanent change in their status and relationships with other personnel.

Crisis management orientation

A major contributor to the dual problem of nursing turnover-retention is the crisis management orientation on the part of the health care organization responsible for direct patient care. Analogies can be drawn between a military organization and a health care organization.

- Most of the training in each is devoted to the action to be taken in a crisis. Procedures are set to define such actions.
- In a crisis situation where the above procedures become appropriate, each member of the unit is expected to carry out the proper steps under the command or scrutiny of a superior, and to do so in a prescribed manner without question.
- The pecking order in a crisis-oriented organization is usually laid out in a rigid hierarchy. In battle, the colonel does what the general says to do. In a hospital, the nurse does what the supervisor or a doctor says to do.

Few would argue that the above conditions constitute the best way to deal efficiently and effectively with a crisis, whether in war or in a health care emergency. Once the crisis orientation is in place, however, there is a tendency to carry over the same management techniques into noncritical situations. It is easier on the "superior" member of the team to keep the relationship on a level where orders are routinely given and taken. To do otherwise requires formal training and practice in participative team-building management techniques. Few health care professionals (nurses, doctors, administrators) receive such educational training in their degree programs. Without such training, it is easier for the perceived superior in the superior-subordinate relationship to remain in the crisis-oriented autocratic role than to make continuing value judgments as to the appropriate leadership style and then switch back and forth.

An orientation toward crisis management may be easier for the superior in a superior-subordinate relationship, but it is difficult for the subordinate who is trying to perform on the job while retaining or building a feeling of self-worth. It is the seeking after the self-fulfilling components of work that serves as the major justification for a nurse's moving from one hospital to another for little or no increase in pay.

Causes and roots of turnover

It should be apparent from the previous pages that the dual problems of nursing shortages and turnover are not simple ones given to simplistic solutions of one dimension. Perhaps the sheer complexity of the problem has kept the research and action focused on the apparent easier remedies; that is, a shortage can be cured by more output from nursing schools, lowered standards, and more effective recruiting. Such actions only disguise the problem. Throughout this book the problem of *turnover-retention* will be addressed, methods will be given and discussed allowing conditions within the hospital and within the nurses to change, and the proven result will be lowered turnover and higher retention. The shortage problem will disappear.

THE IMPACT OF TURNOVER

The effects of nursing turnover are felt throughout the organization whether the consequences are positive or negative in nature. In the positive sense, a certain amount of turnover is needed for renewal of the organization. In the negative direction, excess turnover affects the entire profession of nursing, the cost of health care, and the morale and finances of each institution. Some of the major impacts of turnover are discussed in this section.

Financial

As pointed out earlier in this chapter, the financial aspects of nursing turnover are very sobering. This fact can be demonstrated by means of a hypothetical example (see box on p. 17). Consider a 400-bed hospital with an average occupancy rate of 70%. In general, such an occupancy figure would be lower than ideal, but still not unacceptable to most administrators. Over the course of the year, the hospital would provide about $(400) (.70) (365) = 102,200$ patient days of care. Suppose the hospital has a total of 700 nurses for staffing purposes and that there is a turnover rate of 50% of these nurses, a not uncommon figure. The hospital would be faced with recruiting, hiring, and

A VISUAL PRESENTATION OF SOME COSTS OF TURNOVER

STEP A

400-bed hospital × .70 occupancy rate × 365 days per year = 102,200 patient care days
   per year.

STEP B

700 nurses × .50 turnover rate per year = 350 nurses to be replaced.
350 nurses × $2500 turnover cost per nurse = $875,000 total turnover costs per year.

STEP C

Figure *B* divided by Figure *A* = $8.56 increase in costs per patient care day.

A VISUAL PRESENTATION
OF DECREASED TURNOVER COSTS

STEP A

350 nurses needed per year at a .50 turnover rate − 70 nurses needed per year at a
   .10 rate = 280 nurses difference.

STEP B

280 nurses difference × $2500 turnover costs per nurse = $700,000 savings per year
   in a 400-bed hospital.

training 350 nurses over the course of the year. It has been estimated that turnover costs of one nurse are about $2500. In the hypothesized hospital, the turnover of nurses costs at least (350) (2500) = $875,000 per year. The $875,000 figure alone would add a cost of $875,000/102,200 = $8.56 per patient day. As a novel idea, suppose the money previously spent on the costs associated with turnover were fed directly into the salaries of the retained nurses. What effects might this have on the attitudes of the nurses and on retention?

In the example presented above, the hospital had a 50% turnover rate, necessitating the recruitment of 350 nurses and incurring a cost of $2500 per nurse turnover cost. Suppose the turnover rate could be cut to 10% (see box above). Rather than needing 350 recruited nurses, the hospital would need only 70. This would mean a savings of (350 − 70) nurses times $2500 per nurse, or a savings of $700,000. If these savings could be passed on to the retained nurses, each nurse could be given an average increase of $1000 per year with no extra money being taken from hospital coffers and no rate increase passed on to the consumer.

Other examples could be formulated showing the financial effects of excess nursing turnover. Let it suffice to say that any changes in the turnover rate have a considerable effect on hospital finances.

Turnover also affects the productivity of the nursing unit.

Productivity

Productivity is a word and concept that has been overused to the point that it has almost become a buzzword. Still it is an important and valid issue relevant to nurse retention. Productivity is generally defined or computed as a ratio of output to input or effort, and can be used as a measure of performance at all system levels from the individual worker to the entire organization. Worker productivity and financial performance are highly interrelated. Increased productivity means that an increased workload can be handled by the same number of employees or the same workload can be handled with fewer employees. Either case results in savings regarding the financial responsibilities of the organization.

The health care industry in general and nursing in particular are at a disadvantage in the quest for productivity improvement. A hospital is a highly labor-intensive service organization, and productivity increases are difficult to attain. In service organizations, the two major ways to affect productivity are capital intensity (capital investment in mechanization, better tools, and computers) and more efficient labor practices. Most of a nurse's duties cannot be automated, thus labor practices are of major concern. One "labor practice" amenable to improvement pertains to retention of experienced nurses.

The idea of retention of staff and supervisory nurses has far-reaching and interesting implications. Retention is tied to and has an impact on both the productivity and the financial aspects of a hospital's operation. For instance, consider the impact on the productivity of a nursing unit of a nurse who is retained.

- There is a trained person on the staff who is familiar with the operation of the hospital, with the idiosyncrasies of its personnel, and with its current patients.
- The above familiarities allow the nurse to spend time in patient care rather than in learning the operation of the unit.
- In addition, the nurse who is retained does not take up the time of one or more other unit personnel for orientation, having questions answered, and generally being watched over until he or she is familiar with hospital procedures.
- This trained nurse provides more nursing service than a newly hired nurse, thus yielding more productivity.

- Higher productivity on the part of one nurse, multiplied by several retained nurses, has a tremendous financial impact on the hospital in at least two ways:
  1. Hiring nurses to take up the slack in service caused by a unit staffed by other recently hired nurses does not have to take place. To put it another way, retained and seasoned nurses can provide the same level of services as a greater number of nurses who are less familiar with a specific hospital or unit. Fewer nurses means relatively fewer salary dollars.
  2. Less turnover means less money spent on such expenses as recruiting, severance pay, unemployment benefits, and paperwork changes.

There are financial and productivity aspects of turnover that go far beyond dollars and cents; these are merely the surface. This element of productivity has to do with the attitudes of the retained nurses and their subsequent impact on finances and productivity. These attitudinal variables are explored in virtually all books on management, basic or more advanced. They make a number of points concerning employees in productive enterprises. Chief among these are the following:

- People work better when they believe they have a hand in the decision affecting them.
- People work better when they believe they are making progress toward their own life goals; that is, they are getting close to what they want out of life.
- Managers get better results when they can convince their subordinates that the organization's goals and the subordinate's goals coincide; that is, that the employee can make the best progress toward his or her own goals by helping work toward the organization's goals.

Suppose each staff nurse and supervisory level nurse went to work tomorrow morning knowing that each nurse was working toward the same basic set of goals as he or she was, and was in fact as *supportive* of him or her as this individual was of each of them.

- What would happen to the level of care and the efficiency and effectiveness with which it was carried out?
- What would happen to the nurses' attitudes toward the patients and thus to the patients' morale?
- What would happen to the nurses' attitudes toward each other, toward the hospital in which they work, and toward the nursing profession?
- What would happen to the nurses' use, and watchfulness over the use, of the resources of the hospital?

The positive outcomes generated by answers to these questions would likely lead to untold, albeit intangible, savings. A dollar figure can be determined for a nurse who resigns. A dollar figure can be calculated for the recruitment of a nurse. A more nebulous number can be arrived at for the cost of training the new nurse and covering for lower productivity during the training and familiarization period. It is not likely that a dollar improvement figure resulting from a change in people's *attitudes* can be arrived at; yet common sense tells us it is *there* and that it is important.

Staff maturity

The effects of high turnover are documented in the organization's financial statement and in the quality and quantity of production and services. A high rate of turnover adversely affects the maturity, sophistication, and stability of the organization and of the departments within the organization. Nursing, as a developing profession, is severely handicapped by this phenomenon.

Chris Argyris,[1] identifies seven behavioral tendencies in the process of maturation. Behavior progresses as follows:

1. From a state of being passive to a state of increasing self-directed activity
2. From a state of dependence on others to a state of relative independence
3. From being capable of behaving in only a few ways to being capable of behaving in many ways
4. From having erratic, casual, shallow, quickly dropped interests to a deepening of interests
5. From having a short time perspective to a much broader time perspective
6. From being in a subordinate position to occupying a more equal or superordinate position
7. From a lack of awareness of the self to an awareness and control over one's self

A profession can be examined for maturation utilizing the same criteria.

1. *Passivity versus activity.* Nursing, if not passive, is certainly reactive and responsive rather than proactive and assertive. Comprising the largest number of employees in most health care organizations, nurses are generally the least outspoken, the most predictable and dependable, the most acquiescent, and the most malleable.

2. *Dependence versus independence.* Nursing, by licensure and mandate, works under the direction of the physician. Its procedures require the approval of the medical staff. The philosophy and practice of nursing diagnosis are new; self-evaluating nursing audits have been only recently endorsed. More independent forays are being made (e.g., independent practice, third-party payment to nurses), but these are being made outside of the institution.

3. *Few versus many behaviors*. The stereotypes of the nurse as bedpan carrier or pill pusher have some basis in actual behavior. Without denying the value, worth, and need of physical care, other human needs are too often dealt with only if they can "fit in." Teaching, offering emotional support, family counseling, defining preoperative expectations, recognizing and exploring patient fear and anger: these wait until there is time.

4. *Erratic, shallow, or dropped interests versus deepening interests*. Support systems among nurses are rare. A shared gripe session may occur, but seeking and giving help, counsel, and feedback to one another seldom occurs. The committees on which nurses serve tend to deal with short-term, often superficial issues. It is more common for a nurse to defend "my unit" than to identify with the broader picture of the organizational need and/or the future of the health care delivery system.

5. *Short time versus broader time perspective*. Nursing tends to be crisis oriented. Nurses react more often to issues that are emergent than to those that are important. Today's staffing needs take a higher priority than next year's staffing requirements or than the staff development of present personnel. It is rare indeed that nurses in first-line or middle management take time for long-range planning. And when they do, it is more often met with criticism than with commendation.

6. *Subordinate versus equal or superordinate position*. Nurses who move into nurse management-administration become "the enemy" overnight. Seeking a superordinate position is not valued behavior or ambition. Newly promoted nurses indicate their selection was based on such variables as "there was no one else," "they talked me into it," "it was either me or _____ and I couldn't work for her." There are some nurses seeking equality; unfortunately, too often they are doing so outside of nursing or outside the institution. They have not yet as a group asked for (demanded) equality.

7. *Lack of self-awareness versus self-awareness and self-control*. Frequently the only sense of self for nursing comes in the role of antagonist: nursing versus x-ray, nursing versus the laboratory, nursing versus the physician. A common complaint is that all of the odd jobs fall to nursing: nursing does everything from security to maintenance to cleanup. But nursing lacks a true sense of its own worth, its own description. It does not demonstrate control over itself.

Nursing behaves in a predominately immature way within most hospital (institutional) settings. However, these are the behaviors expected of them by others. Further, it is difficult and actually improper to contemplate new horizons while patient needs go unmet: it is impossible to plan staff development programs with patients and their families clamoring for answers. It is hard to discuss next year's goals when orientation of new personnel takes a quarter of your time. Supportive, caring, confrontive relationships are difficult to maintain when one's peers change from month to month. It takes time for a group of strangers to become a committee. Collegial relationships among nurses are necessary in order to define nursing within an organization, and a mature team is required to present consistently the image that has been defined.

Jack Gibb[10] identifies four stages in group/team development, each focusing on a separate concern that demands resolution. Given the opportunity, a group of individuals begins by dealing with acceptance and membership; the group then develops communication and data flow, norms, and patterns before it moves to the issues of productivity and goal formation; the final step is the struggle toward social control and organization. Consider the impact of a 35 to 50% turnover on this intricate, time-involving process in a unit team, in a committee, in a department. The issue of membership, the initial and most fundamental one, must always be addressed when turnover is high; behavioral symptoms of this issue when unresolved include fear, distrust, legalism, cynicism, suspicion, and conformity. However, when a group has successfully moved through all four stages of group development, behavioral outcomes include coordination, role distribution, shared leadership, interdependence, flexibility, and participative action and structure. Team and/or group development, however, take time. According to George Homans's hypothesis, "people who interact will grow to like each other, assuming they have compatible goals and needs, and this will lead to more interaction (communication), thus establishing a cycle of cohesion."[15] The time (not to mention the *quality* of this time) of group growth does not bode well for a profession with high turnover; it increases the unlikelihood that its work groups can become effectively productive teams.

Morale. Nursing is one of the unique professions whose members predominately select the profession for the purpose of self-actualization, and whose esteem and ego needs are partially met by the title of nurse. A large portion of young people enter schools of nursing in order to provide nurturance and care to the suffering. It is demoralizing when a person embraces a profession for the purpose of fulfilling these higher needs only to have the more basic needs (physiological, safety, and social) poorly met and usually ignored by the organization. The frustration, bitterness, anger, and disillusionment generated by this phenomenon have been aptly researched and described by Marlene Kramer and Constance Baker,[17] and documented by the myriad of exit interviews of burned-out, turned-off nurses.

Productivity, job satisfaction, and staff retention are highly responsive to the morale of the workplace. Herzberg divides job conditions into two factors: maintenance or extrinsic and motivational or intrinsic. His findings indicate that it is the maintenance factors that profoundly affect morale. The factors in the work situation that address the lower order needs of persons, when unsatisfied, cause low morale and high turnover. Porter and Lawler* have defined job satisfaction as being interrelated with reward for job performance, considering both intrinsic and extrinsic rewards as well as the judged equitability of those two reward groups. For the nursing profession, there are too many maintenance factors not being met and too little equitability between intrinsic and extrinsic rewards; hence low morale and high turnover.

It has been said that turnover is infectious. Nurses tend to identify with other nurses; their reference group is one with a professional or cosmopolitan orientation (see section on equity theory in Chapter 4). Consequently, when one nurse leaves an organization, the remaining nurses tend to consider and reexamine their work situation, most often utilizing the criteria of their departed colleague. Suddenly the cherished hopes for change, their expectations for a better tomorrow are revealed in their true perspective: long-term effort and investment that may or may not seem worthwhile. Turnover causes lowered morale, which causes increased turnover. It is a vicious cycle.

Continuity and quality of patient care. Turnover takes its toll also in the quantity and quality of the patient care that it delivers. The new employee is never as productive as the old-timer. Efficiency is, at least in part, a function of familiarity. Routine, procedures, norms, and physical layout take time to learn. Assessing, identifying, demonstrating areas of expertise—expanding into the pool of experts that comprise every unit and department—is a process of mutual examination that takes place over several months. This is the process of determining the degree of fit, both individually and collectively. The development of collegial and superior-subordinate relationships, including the clarification of expectations and assumptions, tends to take an emotional if not actual time priority over patient needs.

Growth (turnover as a positive force) and nongrowth

Total eradication of turnover is impossible. It would also be undesirable. It is, however, possible to stop that turnover that represents waste: waste of dreams, aspirations, and professional goals; waste of time, research, interaction, paperwork, and money; waste through feelings of frustration, failure, disappointment, and mistrust; waste in terms of the loss of quality care, time investment, and follow-through for patients and their families. Some of this waste is demonstrable; significant portions of it are not measurable. All waste reduces the quality of the health care delivery system.

Some turnover has healthy consequences and proactive rationale. A

---

*For a more in-depth examination of motivation and its implications for turnover, see Chapter 4, Motivation (Ref. 15).

proper proportion of turnover is based not so much on a numerical statistic as on the information gathered in exit interviews. It behooves an organization to ask itself, for each reason of turnover that is presented: "Could we have met the need? Could we have harnessed the motivation? Could we have provided the challenge? Is this a productive personnel change for the organization?" The ability to answer these questions honestly rests entirely on the terminating employee's confidence that you want and will accept his or her honest responses.

Turnover allows people to move up, to assume new roles, to try new behaviors. It provides the organization with a fresh mirror for feedback, new insights, new procedures, and new questions. New employees demand explanations about standard operating procedures, help point out the long-accepted inconsistencies, and, when allowed, bring in fresh approaches and new enthusiasm. Stagnation, boredom, lack of investment, and consequently lack of growth occur in a too stable (inert) staff. It is therefore the challenge of nursing leadership and hospital administration to enfuse ongoing challenge and enthusiasm without suffering the waste of high turnover.

Disillusionment

Unlike most other professionals, nurses practice in a work world that is unrelentingly charged with intense human emotions. The burnout syndrome is common to professionals in ongoing, close, and intimate contact with people; such contact is often emotionally difficult to handle. Nurses, by their nature and what they believe they can accomplish in the work setting, often have feelings of inadequacy and frustration as they try to balance institutional demands with patient care needs.

Burnout is, first and foremost, disillusionment. The influence of illusion on human affairs and human activity is intangible but nevertheless present. The presence of a dream is what spurs the individual and certainly the nurse to greater involvement and contribution in the profession. Friction or tension and a certain amount of stress indicate a healthy work situation and provide interest and challenge in a job. When friction does occur, peer support can provide a sense of security. Burnout is the resignation to a lack of power, the perception that no matter what you do or how hard you try, you cannot make a difference in the situation.

Maybe the reason nursing is so misunderstood is that it is so hard to define, even for nurses themselves. Everyone knows what a doctor does or what a lawyer does. Their professional responsibilities are clear and defined in terms of their skill and training. People see lawyers, for example, as representing clients and preparing briefs. However, would the public also see them cleaning up the courtroom if they found it littered or dirty? Most definitely not. Yet nurses are expected to clean up vomit or spills on the floor in an institution because often there is "no one else to do it." Their profession requires that they set their priorities based on who needs them most. Nursing time is frequently allocated to performing tasks that could be handled by others, which would free nurses to utilize their knowledge, skill, and training to attend to other (perhaps higher order) needs of patients.

The nursing shortage is found in the delivery of nursing services rather than in the actual number of nurses. The real problem lies in the definition of nurses' roles. In many institutions nurses are frequently expected to be *ex officio* physicians, pharmacists, housekeepers, transporters, secretaries, messengers, administrators, aides, technicians, dieticians, and social workers. With their free time, if there is any, they are expected to nurse. This misuse and mismanagement of nurses by themselves as well as others results in a lack of motivation and decreased productivity while providing fertile territory for negative factors in the environment to be more important and to take hold.[7]

Another item high on the list for disillusionment with the nursing profession is the economic factor. The women's movement has provided some startling statistics regarding women's pay. In the early 1980s the full-time working woman received 59 cents for every dollar in her male counterpart's paycheck.[13] At that time a woman with 4 years of college earned an average of $13,400, slightly less than a man who had not gone to high school. His take-home pay was about $14,000. The National Research Council in 1981 released a report stating that 70% of men and 54% of women in the labor force were in jobs dominated by members of their own sex. Perhaps the most significant aspect of the conclusion, which applies to nursing, is that the more an occupation is dominated by women the less it pays.

If nursing professionals sometimes find their role confusing, one can imagine what it is like for those in school. The classic nursing text, *Reality Shock: Why Nurses Leave Nursing*, by Marlene Kramer, discussed the dichotomy between what nursing students expect of the profession and what they ultimately discover it to be. The largest number of nurses drop out during their first year and a half, and many others find that hospital work is not for them and seek refuge in a clinic or physician's office. It does not seem that there is one single factor or facet that discourages nurses; rather, it appears to be an endless series of pressures.

The female nurse wants to view herself as cool and competent, in charge of the most difficult and stressful situation, and in her own mind most of the time this is the case. But the real woman beneath the uniform often has trouble coping with her own human frailties and questions her personal presence in this profession. These dilemmas of the "self as nurse" are often evidenced by the types of work-related frustrations experienced and ex-

---

**WORK-RELATED CONCERNS EXPRESSED BY NURSES
THAT ARE RELATED TO ISSUES OF "SELF"**

Understaffing
Too much responsibility too soon for new RNs
Little or no attempt to weed out incompetent help
Weak orientation program
Policies not enforced consistently
Lack of time for patient teaching
Decision making by administration without adequate facts
Decision making by superiors without input from those most familiar with current first-
    hand experience
No positive feedback from supervisors
Decision-making responsibility without authority
No recognition for their abilities as nurses or for significant contributions such as out-
    standing nurse care and innovative ideas
Inadequate rewards for long-term employees

---

pressed by nurses. These frustrations tend not to be characteristics of nursing practice but of management and/or administrative processes. Some specific nurse concerns are listed above.

Enlightened nursing and hospital administrations can make a difference by focusing on these concerns; they can make a difference in the exodus of nurses from hospitals.

Nursing and hospital administrations can create a supportive environment for nurses to realize their personal (intrinsic) fulfillment, which will make nursing a more rewarding career. Administration cannot, however, meet these highly individual and specific needs. Nurses themselves must take action and be responsible in such areas as:

- Accepting the profession for what it is: a profession that is searching for a definition, whose practitioners, if united, can make a difference in the health care delivery system of this country (and beyond)
- Recognizing the problems that nursing is experiencing, and working *within* the profession to change things—that is, being proactive, not reactive
- Being realistic in approaching problems occurring in interpersonal relationships and in supporting peers
- In organizational settings, understanding various elements of an issue, making recommendations for change, offering alternatives and options, being willing to compromise
- Understanding the global picture of health care in our society, being

concerned with all aspects and issues relating to health care, not having tunnel vision as it relates to nursing
- Becoming politically involved, making one's voice count as a nurse and as a consumer of health care

If the administrative staff accepts the tenet that the greatest dissatisfaction in a hospital work setting is not with the work itself but rather with administrative and management practices, then the direction to follow is clear. Nursing and hospital administrations must collaborate with nursing service employees at all levels to develop policies and practices that address nurses' concerns, from innovative scheduling plans to fair and equitable reward systems. Only then will a positive step be effected toward correcting some of the disillusionment nurses express in institutional settings.

Disillusionment in its purest sense is the end of a dream, a personal experience with professional implications.

Prestige of the profession

A female nurse's perception of the profession's prestige can be many-faceted. It depends primarily on how she views herself as a person and then as a woman in a profession that is 98% female. Although there are men within the nursing profession and they are making significant contributions, still nursing equals female. Predominately, moviemakers and television programmers' portrayal of nurses has been as empty-headed, man-chasing females, subservient to physicians and existing only to do menial tasks and to look cute. This has led to the public's perception of hospital nursing as "doctor-nurse games." Nursing as a profession will continue to have problems with prestige and image until the practitioners of the profession cease to think of nursing as (1) a supplementary income to help out the family budget; (2) a second job, less important than the spouse's (even if he has less income); (3) an interim occupation to support you until you can find a husband to take over; and (4) just an 8-hour-a-day job. These demeaning and detrimental concepts must be abandoned, and nursing must be perceived and practiced as a career, a lifelong commitment to a valued, cherished, and respected profession.

Nursing must deal with pluralism in the work force. The proliferation of various types of paramedical workers is causing conflict in terms of licensure, certification, overlapping roles, and scope of practice. Affirmative action programs have involved a greater mix of ethnic groups with varying value systems, which creates the need for change in nursing practice. Nursing leaders must seize the opportunity for input and change, and not wait to react after change has been imposed by those ("others") in power. This can be best illustrated by looking at the past, when nursing provided everything for the care of patients during their hospital stay; now paraprofessionals and technical health care workers are employed to perform highly specialized tasks in the patient's treatment regimen. This has led to the belief by hospital administrators in some areas that if the number of practicing nurses continues to decline, then other workers must be trained to take their place. This has also injected a certain amount of fear and job insecurity into the nurse's perception of the future job market: could hospital administrators decide that if nurses request "too much" (salary, working conditions, fringe benefits), the nurses will be replaced by less-qualified individuals in a purported effort to contain costs?

Nursing continues to demand its proper recognition as a profession making specific contributions in the provision of health care. Different levels of educational preparation in nursing demand coordinated professional attention in order to provide realistic and objective expectations of practice for workers prepared at different levels. Instead of the divisiveness that the different preparations for entry levels into practice have created thus far, creative approaches might be introduced to upgrade the profession and prepare nursing to take its proper place among the other health care professions (medicine, pharmacy, social work, physical therapy, dietetics). One such approach might be to have the BSN (4-year) as the beginning level for professional nursing practice (RN), and have the ADN 2-year programs be the beginning level for technical, vocational, or practical nursing practice (LPN, LVN). Other programs, such as diploma (3-year) and vocational (1-year) programs might then be deleted. The key is assessment, coordination, and consensus.

Nurses by their own inaction have perpetuated the status quo, behaved in an unprofessional manner, overreacted to pertinent health care issues; they have been defensive and made excuses for accepting whatever role others have chosen to assign them. Nurses have left self-actualization and professional growth to other professions; they have in effect ignored new technologies while other groups rushed to embrace the challenge.

It would be an oversight to fail to recognize the part that directors of nursing play in turnover of professional nurses, and further, with the prestige of the profession as a whole. A few nursing directors are creative, participative managers who consider the best interests of their staff and have concern for the future of nursing as their primary goals. These directors do make a difference in turnover rates at their institutions. The sad commentary, however, is that the majority of nursing directors spend much of their time and effort in maintaining the status quo of their position and thus, by implication, the future of those nurses whom they supervise. Too often the female director becomes entrenched in the "queen bee" syndrome, believing that she is unique among nurses and that she should solely identify and align herself with physicians or hospital administrators.

SOME DIRECTIONS FOR MOVING FORWARD

Make a commitment to nursing as a lifelong career.
If there are elements in nursing that need changing, work *within* the profession to change them.
Support other nurses in all areas of nursing.
Build unity in the profession; speak with one voice.
Present nursing as an exciting, altruistic profession whose practitioners are educated, respected, and well paid.
Continue to explore, both personally and in groups, our roots, our contemporary problems, our hopes, and our recommendations for resolution.

The question is: Are the contemporary problems that nursing faces rooted in the lack of definition of what nursing is and how it contributes to the health care delivery system, or is it far more basic than that? Are they the effect of programming and the socialization of women in our society? A strong case can be made for either viewpoint. It is most probable that the problems result from unique combinations of elements from each of the above. Regardless of the causes, definitive actions must be taken and taken soon, because the profession is in trouble (witness retention-turnover statistics). In order to undertake an improvement in the prestige and image of the profession, some symptoms may be treated concomitant with the causes. The most significant measures that can be implemented must be undertaken by nurses themselves. (See list above.)

A CONCEPTUAL CONCLUSION

The terms *effective* and *efficient* have over the past several decades become increasingly useful as means of describing organizational operations and activities. They have been used to enhance the crucial planning and evaluation phases of organizational life. Recently the two concepts have been applied to managerial styles and behaviors vis-à-vis the carrying out of managerial responsibilities. It is our perspective that these terms directly apply to the problems of (1) the retention of nurses in hospital settings and (2) the present developmental stage of the nursing profession. Additionally, we believe that these two problems are so intricately intertwined that efforts toward resolution of either or both will have profound effects on the total field of health care (see Kurt Lewin, Field Theory). It is beyond the scope of this book to focus continually on this relationship; it has, however, been addressed in the preceding pages. We have not developed the premise in our efforts here, but we do hope that the implications will be further considered (especially by the profession). Earlier in the chapter we referred to three time periods in the development of nursing. Perhaps our book will be a part of heralding the fourth period in nursing history.

Efficiency and effectiveness defined

In the meantime, to demonstrate how effectiveness and efficiency apply to the retention of nurses, we must begin with adequate definitions of each. *Efficiency* refers to the selection and utilization of the most current, practical, proven technologies, methodologies, programs, and equipment available to accomplish the tasks of the organization. The degree to which organizations (and their administrative leadership) are "doing *things* right" determines their degree of efficiency. Examples of efficiency-related mechanisms include hospital room furniture, operating room equipment, computer information systems, computer programs, organization design, in-house management development activities, recruitment strategies, personnel policies and procedures, time-sharing, flexible scheduling options, tax programs, inventory systems, investment strategies, community activities, budgeting programs, performance appraisal systems, and promotion plans. The key to efficiency is objective tools that are put in place to carry out the major organizational activities necessary to accomplish the organizational objectives. It is the "volume and quality of the output relative to the resource inputs."[8] An efficient manager is one who recognizes the major managerial functions and who then consistently seeks mechanisms to carry out these functions. Such mechanisms may include participative decision making, delegation, a flexible and consistent personal style, an office, regular meetings, written and verbal communication strategies, and interaction with and among subordinates, peers, superiors.

Effectiveness is a broader concept both organizationally and generically. *Effectiveness* refers to how the mechanisms of efficiency are implemented. According to Peter Drucker, it is the result of doing the right *thing* in relation to organizational objectives and needs. Effectiveness rests on the choices made, the organization's short-range objectives, and its human systems. The degree to which an organization is effective is based on three variables:

1. Organizational efficiency
2. Equilibrium in the social-interpersonal subsystem
3. Anticipating and preparing for change (and the future)[8]

An effective manager is one who carries out his or her responsibilities according to three criteria:

1. Efficiency
2. People (groups and individuals) needs
3. Impact on present and future

The effective manager usually struggles with but is willing to make decisions based on these criteria, and can do so without creating excessive tension and stress (to organizational effectiveness).

...and the retention of nurses

It is our hypothesis that hospital efforts toward nurse retention have primarily focused on strategies encompassed within the definitions of efficiency. We believe that both organizational policies and programs and individual administrator-manager activities have been implemented as they affect efficiency. We recognize the far-reaching contributions of concepts that many hospitals have installed, such as the career ladder, matrix organizations, recruitment specialists and activities, broadly based management input interventions, increased benefits in terms of organizational efficiency. However, it is unlikely that these mechanisms will have the lasting impact being sought: the ongoing retention of nurses. The profession of nursing too has fallen victim to (and prisoner of) the simplistic notions of generating the "proper" mechanisms to become professional, to develop as a profession, and to solve problems. This orientation toward efficiency has as a result greatly inhibited the profession's ability to contribute significantly to the problem of retention.

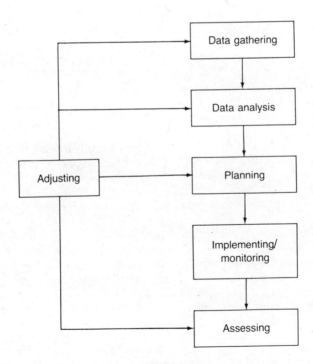

FIG. 1-1
Nurse retention program.

Hospital administrators, organizational actions, and the nursing profession must now consider effectiveness. They must initiate the *process* rather than gather additional tools and techniques. Effectiveness in terms of nurse retention can be accomplished by the normative process of asking three questions: Where are we? Where do we want to be? How do we get from where we are to where we want to be? These questions translate into the process depicted in Fig. 1-1. But it is more far-reaching than this process. Effectiveness must mean modeling and involving all levels and members of the organization; it must include allowing and resolving conflict; it must value and consider individual differences and input; and most importantly, effectiveness means one must constantly look at one's *self*—interpersonal style, communication methods, value system, orientation toward humanity and people, view of and hopes for the future.

To solve the nurse retention problem, the nursing profession and each separate organization must be willing to commit themselves to the process of *E + E* (efficiency plus effectiveness).

Our book reflects our commitment to this premise. It also reflects our commitment to professional nursing and to organizational productivity. In terms of hospitals and health, they are inseparable.

REFERENCES AND ADDITIONAL READINGS

1. Argyris, C.: Personal versus organizational goals, Yale Scientific **34**(1):40-50, Feb. 1960.
2. Bayer, A.E.: Nurse supply: it's better than we thought, Mod. Hosp. **109**(1): 75-79, 1967.
3. Bays, K.D.: Capsule, J. Nurs. Admin. **21**(9):16, Sept. 1981.
4. Brown, E.L.: Nursing for the future, New York, 1948, Russell Sage Foundation.
5. Cathcart, H.R.: Nursing commission issues preliminary report, Hospitals **9**:23-24, Sept. 16, 1981.
6. Conerley, P.K.: Attitudes of RN's in northwest Florida toward continuing education, masters thesis, The University of West Florida, Pensacola, 1974.
7. Curtin, L.: A shortage of nurses—or the sabotage, editorial, Super. Nurse **12**(4): 7, April 1981.
8. Duncan, W.J.: Organizational behavior, ed. 2, Boston, 1981, Houghton-Mifflin Co.
9. Florence Nightingale, rebel with a cause, booklet reprinted from RN Magazine (editorial), May 1970.
10. Gibb, J.: Climate for trust formation. In Bradford, L.P., Gibb, J.R., and Benne, K.D., editors: T-Group theory and laboratory method, New York, 1964, John Wiley & Sons, Inc.
11. Goldmark, J.: Nursing and nursing education in the United States, New York, 1923, The Macmillan Co.
12. Graves, H.H.: Survival in the system, J. Nurs. Admin. **3**(4):26-31, July-Aug. 1973.
13. Green, L.: The pay gap: why do women earn 59¢ for every dollar a man makes? Chicago Sun-Times (Living, Section 4), pp. 8-9, Oct. 25, 1981.

14. Grissum, M., and Speagler, C.: Woman power and health care, Boston, 1976, Little, Brown and Co.
15. Homans, G.C.: The human group, New York, 1950, Harcourt, Brace.
16. Jensen, D.M.: A history of nursing, St. Louis, 1943, The C.V. Mosby Co.
17. Kramer, M., and Baker, C.: The exodus: can we prevent it? J. Nurs. Admin. 1(3): 15-30, Nov.-Dec. 1971.
18. Likert, R.: The human organization: its management and value, New York, 1967, McGraw-Hill Book Co.
19. Price, J.L.: The study of turnover, Ames, 1977, The Iowa University Press.
20. Roseman, E.: Managing employee turnover, New York, 1981, Amacom.
21. Temperley, S.R.: Personnel planning and occupational choice, London, 1974, George Allen & Unwin, Ltd.

2

THE ENTRY PROCESS AND ITS CONSEQUENCES

HUMAN RESOURCE PLANNING
  Definition
  Process
  Conceptual framework
  Critical issues and practical implications
  Assessment questions
RECRUITMENT
  Definition
  Process
  Conceptual framework
  Critical issues and practical implications
  Assessment questions
SELECTION
  Definition
  Process
  Conceptual framework
  Critical issues and practical implications
  Assessment questions
PLACEMENT
  Definition
  Process
  Conceptual framework
  Critical issues and practical implications
  Assessment questions
ORIENTATION
  Definition
  Process
  Conceptual framework
A CONCEPTUAL CONCLUSION

Many cases of turnover have their roots in the entry process. Seeds for termination have been sown before the employee reaches the actual work area. Ineffective, inefficient practices and behaviors in this early phase of the employee life cycle contribute to undermine the new employee's enthusiasm, interest, and intention to stay. Nursing units demand that their vacant positions be filled and that they receive their full quota of employees without recognizing changes in organizational goals, community needs, employee growth and sophistication, and technical advances. Personnel departments judge their recruitment successes by volume. Applicants are selected whose turnover predictability is offset by the need to hire someone, to do something. When the applicant's chosen interest area is unavailable, alternative placement sacrifices efficiency, effectiveness, and job satisfaction because, after all, nursing is nursing. Orientation has become so standardized, so routinized, that it is frankly nonfunctional. Motions are gone through with little variation in actors, topic, or emotional involvement.

Chapter 2 will examine the following five steps in the entry process: employee planning, recruitment, selection, placement, and orientation. Each step will be defined in terms of its purpose/intent, its conceptual framework, its critical issues, and its practical implications. Each section will conclude with a questionnaire that can be utilized as an organizational, departmental, or individual assessment tool; as a group these questionnaires may serve as a beginning climate survey instrument.*†

HUMAN RESOURCE PLANNING
Definition

The human resource plan is the people budget of the organization. It represents, in terms of personnel, the goals and objectives of the organization. It is a "people plan" listing in detail the resources (actual and estimated) to be assigned to a particular service, division, or project for a given future time period. It identifies and underlines current organizational emphasis, suggests and demonstrates areas of organizational weakness, and predicts and implies areas of high (and low) productivity and performance.

Process

The process of human resource planning has political, economic, legal, community, technical, organizational, and social ramifications. It is a logical, interactive, and dynamic organization process. The allocation of human re-

---

Note: The undertaking of a broad, other person–involving climate survey carries with it the obligation to utilize acquired data for growth, change, feedback. Failure to do so will result in greater job dissatisfaction and higher turnover.
†See Chapter 8 for a more in-depth discussion of survey research implications, methodology, and impact.

sources affects day-to-day staffing, staff development, recruitment, program planning, service provision and thus purchasing, capital improvement, and public relations. Consequently, the effective human resource planning process includes input from many disciplines, interest groups, and individuals. Parameters are outlined by accrediting bodies (JCAH, NLN) and by third-party paying agencies (e.g., Medicare, Blue Cross/Blue Shield) for minimum requirements. However, to leave the task of human resource planning to "corporate staff specialists who do wonderful things with numbers but have limited understanding of personnel management at the operating unit level" may result in "an elegant treatment of data based on unrealistic assumptions."[6] The process of human resource planning is representative, indicative, and supportive of the organization's behavior and goals.

There are dynamic forces, both internal and external, that impact on the organization, necessitating changes in the utilization of, development of, and search for human resources. Planning is therefore an ongoing task: noting and recording changes, gathering data, and seeking input. This is not to imply that the human resource plan should be changed daily; that would be farcical. It is necessary, however, for organizations to update, reexamine, and change their human resource budget on an annual (quarterly or semiannually when the organizational environment is rapidly changing) basis. Bruce Coleman[2] suggests six formal steps in the decision-making process for employment planning.

Step 1: Examine organizational goals and objectives
Step 2: Identify gross employee requirements
Step 3: Conduct employee inventory
Step 4: Examine employee programs
Step 5: Compute net employee requirement

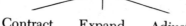

Step 6: Contract   Expand   Adjust

Step 1 takes into consideration not only the mission statement of the organization, but also the direction or program to be emphasized in the coming year. It recognizes changes in competition, community, technology, and the business (professional) environment. The wise planner allows for both stated and understood organization goals, those that are given lip service as well as those that demand significant time and resource allocation.

Step 2 suggests an openness to creativity and innovations as well as practicality and awareness of need. It assumes a thought process of "if we want to do this, we require this many people," rather than "we have these people, therefore we can do this." The gross employee requirement does not concern itself with numbers alone but with qualities, qualifications, education, experience, and aspirations as well.

Step 3 consists of an inventory involving assessment of human resources, and an identification and awareness of personnel wealth. Also, beyond simply supplying numbers, this step considers and records staff growth and maturation, continuing education participation, new interests, and accomplishments.

Step 4 involves an additional facet of the employee inventory. It involves a thorough investigation of internal staff development, identifying those persons who have been involved in premanagement training or who have been in assistant roles, or those who have developed beyond their present role. It is an attempt to promote from within, to provide new challenges to present employees.

Step 5 is a process of matching, of looking for similarities; it results in identification of variance, imbalance, or fit. This step involves synthesizing all acquired data and yielding a picture of unmet human resource requirements. Step 5 results in final decisions: to contract, to expand, to adjust, and where? *Contraction* suggests termination, early retirement, layoff, nonreplacement. *Expansion* refers to hiring, promoting, developing, adding. *Adjustments* are often not considered but include flextime, half shifts, changing departments, combining units, demotions, and a wide variety of further creative options.

The value and impact of each step in this process is assumed. The appropriateness of the resultant decision is directly proportional to the quality and quantity of input received. As with all decisions, it is possible to conduct human resource planning (a) by oneself with one's own data, (b) gathering data from individuals to help one decide, (c) sharing problems with individuals to gather their input, (d) collecting a group for the sake of soliciting input, and (e) allowing an appropriate group to make the decision.[18] Borrowing from Vroom and Yetton, it may be wise for hospital human resource planners to question themselves in light of the retention of professional nurses:

1. Is there a quality requirement to this decision such that one choice may increase turnover?
2. Do I know which choices will increase retention among present staff?
3. Is the above information available in one place?
4. If the professional nurses do not accept (value) my plan, is it implementable?
5. If I develop the staffing plan by myself, will the professional nurses accept it?
6. Do the professional nurses share the organizational goals?
7. If I decide the wrong way, is higher turnover likely?

Acceptance of decisions is rarely an issue with hospital nursing personnel. However, noninvolvement in decisions is a major cause of turnover. Quality of staffing and staff development is another major factor in turnover. Rarely have data on nursing needs and wants been retained "in one place" in an organization. The answers to Vroom and Yetton's modified questions tend to encourage greater nurse involvement in the human resource planning of the organization. Perhaps, though, it all hinges on the answer to question 6. Do you believe that the professional nurse shares in the organization's goals?

Conceptual framework

Expanding on James's theory,[9] human resource planning may be said to be a function of the formation of an employee coalition through negotiation, communication, and problem solving in order to implement organization goals and objectives optimally (see Fig. 2-1).

The term *coalition* addresses the fluidity, changing nature, and blending of forces that comprise the work force of an organization. Professional philosophies, individual interests, departmental priorities, organization history, and community pressure are among the forces that impact on this coalition. Human resource planning emphasizes the *formation* of such a coalition, the dis-

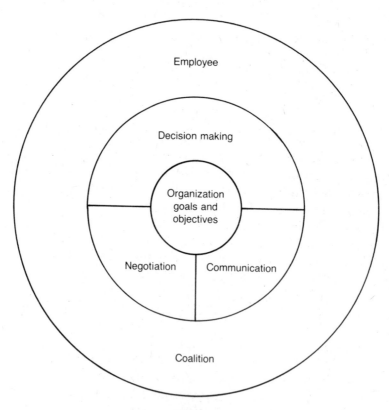

FIG. 2-1
Human resource planning.

cussing, working, compromising, conflicting, helping, and confronting to reach a consensus agreement representing the best way to achieve corporate goals. This "best way" remains totally relevant and receives support and committed effort only for the life of this coalition (another reason high turnover is so costly). The effectiveness of the plan, the uniformity with which it is operationalized, and the support it receives are largely measurable by the strength and completeness of negotiation, communication, and decision making.

The process of negotiating allows each person and each department to present themselves and to explain, elaborate, identify, and defend their strengths, desires, and needs in light of the organization goals. It is a time for mutual exploration and searching for common ground: Does the coalition offer the individual and group what they need? Does the coalition need and/or want what the individual and group are willing to offer? Each individual and each department actively, passively, and sometimes passive-aggressively, negotiate for a position, and for recognition within the coalition. Communication necessarily accompanies negotiation. Within the coalition there is an attempt to speak and listen, to give and receive, to question and answer, to argue and agree in order to arrive at common understandings. Decision making is the product of communication and negotiation. The coalition, this particular joining of forces, decides on required human resources and the allocation of same.

Critical issues and practical implications

Based on the preceding theoretical constructs, critical issues for proactive human resource planning are evident.

Organizational goals. Organization goals must be known and understood by the employees in order for these goals to be attained. Whether they are lofty or plebeian, they must be clarified, publicized, and translated into measurable standards. The degree to which the stated organization objective is believed to be the actual objective is an accurate predictor of human resource commitment and productivity. When the organization goal encompasses the professional and personal goals of its employees, the results are personnel retention, advancement, and satisfaction.

Behaviors. Behavior that is acceptable, prescribed, and rewarded will be identified and mirrored in human resource planning. An organization run by rigid policies and procedures will likely produce a human resource plan mathematically; an organization with loose, barely existing policies and procedures will likely have neither a formal plan nor a usual planning process. The more familiar a multidisciplinary planning meeting, the more likely a group composed of various professional members can efficiently and effectively agree on the utilization of its human resources. Further, groups that are accustomed to utilizing bounded rationality, to taking the first reasonable solution, are not likely to be highly creative or innovative. Commitment to the organization goals and support of human resource plans are habitual; belief and trust in co-workers is either consistently present or absent.

Belief and values. Of particular importance to the human resource planner(s) is the value of each employee or of various employees. When one employee is expendable and another is not, emphasis is often placed on the well-being of the "nonexpendable person." An understanding of personal behaviors and attitudes that are laudable is imperative to proper planning. It is necessary to understand which is the priority issue: the job content (what is done) or the job process (how things are done).

Flexibility. Utilization of and planning for human resources is both a day-to-day and a long-range effort. Changes in industry direction as well as large-scale resignations are conditions the plan must consider. Careful planning recognizes the needs of the fledgling employee, the maturing staff member, and the person who is retiring. An openness to and awareness of these unique needs, strengths, and limitations, combined with considerable creativity and sensitivity make up the ongoing challenge of human resource planning.

Outcomes. A proactive human resource plan encompasses, interprets, and is consistent with the organization's goals and objectives. As is appropriate to the leadership milieu, the planner utilizes the coalition of present employees to assess and redefine its membership needs. Recognizing the need for consistent interpretation of the plan and its cooperative implementation, the planner involves and communicates with appropriate persons. Finally, a realistic, supported human resource plan is the foundation for productivity.

Assessment questions

For the organization:

1. Is the organization's mission statement in writing?
2. Is the organization's mission statement routinely shared with new employees?
3. Are the organization's annual goals publicized? How?
4. Is a general, long-range (5-year, 10-year, 20-year) plan available to staff?
5. Is input sought from each department (person) for planning?
6. Is approval sought for plans before adoption?
7. What do the employees say is the organization's mission, its annual goals?
8. What does the community perceive to be the organization's mission, its goals?
9. Do policies and procedures reflect the organization's goals?
10. How are the various departments ranked according to their organization value? Individuals' ranking within their departments?

11. Which is reinforced as a rule: creativity or conformity?
12. How are interdisciplinary conflicts handled?
13. How is staff growth recognized and/or rewarded?
14. What is the purpose of the staff development department? How is it used?
15. What are the criteria for recognition?
16. What do employees see as criteria for recognition?

For the individual departments:
1. Do we record individual staff contributions? Do we publicize them?
2. Do we record ongoing staff education? Publicize?
3. Do we reinforce employees trying out new behaviors, new roles?
4. Are committees representative of all staff orientations?
5. Do employees know which performance will be rewarded?
6. How do we foster interdepartmental discussion? Planning? Cooperative effort?

For the individual:
1. How am I changing?
2. Who knows I am changing?
3. What are my career goals?
4. What job positions are available now?
5. What do I want to try next?
6. How (and for what) do I want rewards?
7. Do I understand the organization's goals? The annual emphasis?
8. Do I know where I belong in (fit into) these organization goals?
9. How in tune are my goals with the organization's goals?
10. What skills that I can develop will the organization need next year? In 2 years?
11. What am I willing to do to remain a part of this organization?
12. Am I willing to fight for what I think is fair and right in order to feel satisfied with remaining here?

RECRUITMENT
Definition

The function of recruitment is the first step in implementing the human resource plan. Closely related to and often combined with selection, it is the process whereby an organization attracts appropriately qualified job applicants. It is a set of activities designed to induce sufficient numbers of selectively described persons to seek employment with the organization in order to enable the organization to attain its goals effectively. Recruitment efforts communicate to the outside world the current conditions, goals, philosophies, and values of the organization.

Process

The art of recruitment has become a vocation of its own, requiring a specific set of skills, aptitudes, and experience. Prototypes of effective recruiters may be found in the traveling medicine man and the circus barker: "Come one, come all, try my famous . . ." or "See the one and only. . . ." As long as recruitment efforts were evaluated by volume of response alone, these same practices were applicable. As recruiters began to be utilized by the professions, however, emphasis changed from volume of response to appropriateness of respondents. It is therefore essential that the recruiter be (1) thoroughly knowledgeable regarding the organization's goals, mission, and philosophy, as well as (2) intimately aware of the reality and the nuances of the human relations plan.

The policies and procedures of the organization and of the department are important considerations in the early phases of the recruiting process. Common understanding regarding internal promotion, promotion on the same unit, promotions to another unit, utilizing completed education (e.g., nurse's assistant to registered nurse), and the ramifications of these practices must be worked out with significant persons within the organization and the specific department. Values and policies concerning related employees (e.g., sisters) working on the same unit provide relevant data.

The human resource plan, modified by selected organization policies and practices, provides the recruiter with the personnel requirements. The recruiter is then faced with the task of finding applicants with the identified credentials and characteristics, and then obtaining their interest and application. The more specific the requirements, the more arduous the task. Simply seeking nurses is quite different from soliciting for an experienced intensive care, geriatric, pediatric, infection control, or supervisory nurse. Complying with the spirit of the organization, remaining within the bounds of the human resource plan, allowing for intelligence and self-direction in the applicant, and successfully introducing new people into departments are components that demand creativity, ingenuity, and integrity on the part of the recruiter.

Nurses are everywhere. They are in doctor's offices, in the PTA, working at the hospital down the street, retired from practice, working at the supermarket, working across the country, enrolled in higher education. They are fulfilled and challenged as well as bored and undervalued. Nurses may be recruited through public and private employment offices; by advertising in local papers or trade journals or on the radio and television; through schools and universities; through unions; by referral from past and present employees; by recommendation of patients or patients' families; and by means of good fortune (the unsolicited applicant).

The source of recruits has ramifications for the organization, the department, and the industry. Seeking nonnursing nurses brings with it the onus of reteaching, demands a specialized orientation, and tends to result in greater expenditures in time and effort by the organization. However, the disadvantages can be offset if the nurse is retained in the work force for another 5 to 10 years.

Recruiting from schools of nursing involves additional requirements: longer orientation, flexibility, tolerance, and an existing contingent of more sophisticated personnel. When recruits are brought in from out of town or out of state, the recruiting costs are higher and the new employee has personal as well as professional adjustments to make. In-house recruiting may result in wider organization disruption because each position filled creates another opening. Choosing the source of recruits is a function of the qualifications of required applicants in combination with resources of the organization, urgency of the need, and community resources. In equation form:

$$\text{Recruitment source} = f\left(\frac{\text{Desired qualifications}}{\substack{\text{Organization's resources} + \text{Urgency} + \\ \text{Community resources}}}\right)$$

For example, an organization that is located in a geographic area without a college or university and desires applicants with advanced educational degrees must seek recruits from out of the city or state, often utilizing more organizational resources and frequently taking more time.

Recent research by Breaugh[1] identified variation in performance related to the recruitment source. Examining such variables as work quality, quantity, dependability, job knowledge, absenteeism, job involvement, and supervisory satisfaction, his results prove significant for recruiters. Employees recruited through college placement offices were found to be inferior in performance quality and dependability, lower in job involvement, and less satisfied with supervision than recruits from other sources. Persons recruited through newspaper advertising were absent from work twice as often as those recruited from any other source. "Taken as a whole, these results demonstrated that college placement offices and newspaper advertisements were poorer sources of employees than were journal/convention advertisements and self-initiated contacts."[1]

Successful recruiting depends primarily on knowing where to look for people and how to attract their attention. It is based on knowledge, awareness, and research regarding media following and journal readership, as well as skillful, creative, and sometimes ingenious methods of presenting the organization and its personnel needs. Recruitment, like any other aspect of organizational functioning, is judged by its efficiency and effectiveness. Consequently, huge numbers of inappropriate applications represent failure of the recruiting effort. The recruitment officer's worth is no longer equated with the volume of paper that results from his or her endeavors. Overqualified, underqualified, and inappropriate applications frequently result from misrepresentation of, or misleading or inaccurate portrayal of the organization and/or the job requirements.

A current fad in nurse recruiting is the offering of bounties, bonuses, and material inducements to gain applications. The practice seems as appropriate to the process of interesting committed professionals as would be a practice of offering $50 to test-drive a Rolls Royce: ridiculous, unprofessional, and degrading. Dean Wagner of the School of Nursing, University of Wisconsin in Eau Claire, says: "Maybe I'm overreacting, but I can't shed a feeling that bounties reduce nurses to the status of slaves, animal pelts, or outlaws."[19] Fortunately, some health care institutions are putting their "bounties" into rewards that are more consistent with their overall purpose and philosophy; monies are being spent on relocation allowances, professional seminars and memberships, tuition reimbursement, child care, paid parking, flexible shifts, modified schedules, and split jobs.

An advertisement, that is an announcement regarding job openings, presents at best a sketchy idea of what is required. After gaining the attention of interested parties, it is necessary to elaborate, refine, and complete the picture for persons who respond. Accurate job descriptions and behavioral expectations may dull some interest initially, but will assure greater job satisfaction later as well as serve the needs of both the applicant and the organization. Maintaining the enthusiasm of the applicant is a function of the recruiting staff's abilities to follow through, their skill in providing credible answers to questions, and the genuineness of their interest in the candidate.

It is worthwhile to note here the dilemma of the recruiter. Recruiters have much of the education, philosophy, orientation, beliefs, and values of the employment counselor. As such, it is appropriate to suggest to certain inquirers that they not seek employment with a particular organization. On occasion, it would be expedient to suggest there is an appropriate vacancy at a competing facility. This kind of behavior, if carried out, is apt to be disapproved by one's administration. The struggle is waged between what is the best and what is expected and rewarded. A second version of this dilemma is faced by applicants whose desires and/or aspirations do not fit the organization's needs, yet their past experience does. Or their specific skills (such as GI nursing) are less important than their general qualities (medical surgical nursing). Thus the conflict: what is best for the applicant versus what is expedient for the organization. Networking among recruiters, sharing needs and resources, is one approach to more elegant treatment of these problems. Unfortunately, at this time, competition is more the norm than is collaboration.

The recruitment phase of human resource utilization is a process of working to match and complement two sets of preferences: one on the part of the individual, the other on the part of the organization. After interest has been

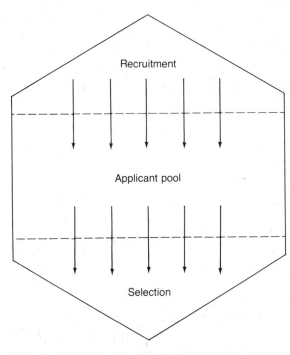

FIG. 2-2
Employment process.

developed, inquiries answered, qualified persons identified and encouraged, and applications presented, the task of recruitment is completed.

Conceptual framework

The process of recruitment may be viewed as the growth of an idea. The seed of the idea (i.e., we need personnel) is defined, refined, elaborated, described, presented, explained, qualified, communicated, and passed on. It has been defined as the positive side of the employment process.[3] It is the act of gathering many interested parties, of identifying varied and new approaches to fulfilling the requirements of the human resources plan. The negative portion of the employment process (selection) is the process of eliminating applicants, choosing preferred candidates. The two halves of the process may be pictured as a hexagon (see Fig. 2-2).

Recruitment by itself consists of four phases: generation, announcement, elaboration, negotiation (see Fig. 2-3). The applicant pool represents the common ground between recruitment and selection.

Generation. The generation phase of recruitment represents a time for data gathering, for creativity and assessment, for flexibility in examining the organization's personnel needs and desires. This includes examination of past re-

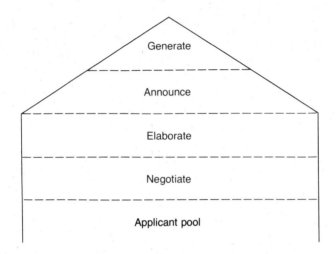

FIG. 2-3
Steps in recruitment.

cruitment successes and failures, interaction, communication, and decision making with present employees. This is the time for self-examination: Is the task proactive or reactive? Are there employee needs or simply vacant positions?

Announcement. The phase of announcement represents "casting bread upon the waters," presenting one's requirements to a critical, significant public. Criteria for judging an applicant's presentation are also applicable for assessing the organization's announcement; important among these are professionalism, efficiency, conciseness, style, confidence, poise, honesty, and consistency. As the effects of the announcement are expected to cause echoes and reverberations, this phase broadens the scope and content of the generated ideas. Considering the importance of attracting appropriate applicants, placement and timing of the announcement are significant. Echoes that consist of meaningless noise are futile.

Elaboration. Responsiveness characterizes the elaboration phase. The recruitment staff will be asked to clarify, defend, explain, and further describe the job requirements, atmosphere, and benefits. Wanous suggests that "individuals possessing more complete information will not be likely to consider jobs that do not match their needs. Thus, those individuals who choose to join the organization will be more satisfied with their jobs than will individuals who possessed less complete and less accurate information."[1]

Although the numbers of interested parties may diminish through this stage, the perspective possessed by the appropriate candidate is expanded.

Negotiation. The next stage involves bargaining, arranging, and exploring ways to meet the needs of both parties. It is a time of following through with discussions and of clarifying the expectations of both organization and individual to determine possible fit. "In many cases, maintaining a labor supply is a matter of one-on-one negotiations with potential employees."[13]

Applicant pool. The contribution to the applicant pool by the recruiter consists of (1) completed applications and (2) thorough transfer of data to those persons involved in the selection portion. This is a time of vulnerability, as often it is here that enthusiasm wanes and positive feelings for the organization may be lost in the transfer of a spokesperson. All employee planning and recruitment efforts now depend on high-caliber selection principles and behaviors.

Critical issues and practical implications

Successful recruitment resulting in retained employees is significantly influenced by the following critical issues. Some of these issues suggest approaches useful to the recruiters, some identify areas for organizational change, and others merely indicate problems.

The organization. Many aspects of the recruiting organization influence the task: its size, location, age, policies, specialties, benefits package, affiliations with educational institutions, professional reputation, programs, administrator, board of directors, community reputation, parking facilities, and cafeteria. It is advisable for the recruiter to emphasize the positive aspects of the organization; for example, small but intimate or multifaceted and challenging. It may also be a sensible strategy for an organization to put its bonus and bounty monies into modifying the negative aspects of its situation and/or reputation; for example, free and secure parking, on-site child care center, nurses serving on planning committees. Organizations make or imply many promises through their advertising campaigns. Retention is impossible if those promises are not both explicitly and implicitly kept. Further, persons wined and dined before employment and taken for granted after hiring are not likely to remain with the organization for long periods of time. For optimum retention purposes, it is important that the organization establish a relationship with its personnel that is consistent.

The personnel. An organization derives its reputation from its structure, services, philosophy, policies, personnel, and clients. The recruiting agent represents the first official contact for potential employees. The value and importance that the organization places in the function of recruiting will be reflected in the sophistication, professionalism, and integrity with which the task is performed.

Present employees are excellent recruiters in terms of job satisfaction and retention. Consequently, it is worthwhile to involve current personnel in recruitment efforts and to keep them advised of job openings and growth opportunities. Should present staff members indicate reluctance to recruit friends, acquaintances, and colleagues, the source of this reluctance is an important change area for the organization.

Satisfied clients are another significant factor in recruitment. They tend to create and support the community image of "the nurses at _____ hospital." This image and reputation can be a drawing card or a repellent for the organization.

The environment. The community environment within which the health care institution is located, as well as the very uncertain professional environment of health care, affect the facility's ability to recruit appropriate personnel. A community that has no higher education programs in nursing requires more elaborate, widespread time- and money-consuming efforts to fill top positions. In this situation, community assets and liabilities are a factor in successful recruitment. The instability crisis in nursing at present is a potent factor in recruitment. The nursing shortage (real or imagined) is such that demand exceeds supply. Consequently, more nurses are job-shopping, thus undermining the stability of the organization. The fluidity of nurses and the paucity of tenured staff have created staffing shortages, lessened the quality of care, diminished organizational reputation, and increased the need for recruitment.

The ethics. As stated earlier, recruitment had its beginning with the circus barker or the traveling medicine man. The advantage these persons had over the recruiter is that they could leave town. False recruiting promises haunt recruiters. Shady behavior is aptly labeled in the community. Stealing competitors' employees is repaid in kind. Less than professional actions result in less than professional recruits. The ends and the means of recruitment will be consonant.

The measurement. The recruitment effort is judged satisfactory when it results in satisfied employees who continue with the organization, when the effort is proactive and future oriented instead of reactive and crisis oriented. It is successful when it involves others; when it reflects and puts into operation the organization's goals; when it is time efficient, cost effective, and personally satisfying for potential and actual employees. Achieving these very high standards is not only the result of meritorious effort; it is a direct outcome of feedback, quality control, and research on the part of the recruiters. Ongoing assessment and investigation into successes and failures is imperative to the proper performance of the recruitment function.

Assessment questions

For the organization:
1. What is the organization's reputation in the community?
2. What are the recruitment strengths?
3. What are the recruitment liabilities?

4. How is the recruiter viewed by colleagues, staff, and administration?
5. What is the recruitment/retention ratio?
6. What recruitment behaviors are rewarded? Expected?
7. What are the causes of lost recruits?
8. How are potential employees treated differently from present staff members?
9. Are policies and procedures favorable to retention or turnover?
10. (a) To what length would the organization go to recruit qualified personnel?
    (b) Does this differ (and how) for different levels and qualifications of recruits?
11. Have recruitment controls and standards been established? How are they monitored?

For the recruiter:
1. Who is supportive of recruitment efforts?
2. Are present employees involved?
3. From where have successes come?
4. From where have failures come?
5. How do you perceive and project your role; your organization?
6. How do you measure success?

SELECTION
Definition

Selection is a process of choosing, of declaring a preference, of identifying those applicants who represent the best fit between the organization's goals and the individual's needs. It is the practice of investigating, interrogating, and interpreting. The art and science of selection involve a composite of skills: risk taking, accurate assessment, tabulations of data, communication abilities, objectivity, and humanity. Selection assumes knowledge of the organization, its jobs, its philosophy and mission, and its atmosphere. The selection process is one of reduction, that is, diminishing the number of candidates and potential employees. The person charged with the role of selection has a dual concern: control and responsibility. "One major element of control which an organization possesses is the ability to choose its employees."[17] The final act of selection gives up that control at the same time it commits the organization to the individual applicant.

Process

A set of behaviors and activities that is designed to identify favored candidates is assumed to be based on identified, measurable criteria. The specificity and/or flexibility of the criteria greatly affect the ease and satisfaction of the task. Seeking any RN who will work nights is vastly different from searching for an RN who will be a functioning member of the cardiac rehabilitation team. Likewise "we need RNs" calls for different behaviors than "we need an experienced psychiatric nurse."

In order to select for retention, behavioral criteria must be envisioned, described, and identified. This process was broadly begun in human resource planning and elaborated on during recruitment. It is at this stage necessary to hone the criteria, that is, to delineate more clearly the characteristics and qualities of the ideal candidate. Typically this skill is not well defined in nursing. As a rule they take what they can get.

The identification of proper selection criteria begins with a clear operational definition of what the chosen applicant will be expected to do, that is, a behavioral job description. Based on the job description, past employee performance, and knowledge of the system, it is possible to identify certain criteria that will predict positive performance and adjustment. These criteria become the basis for future decision making. Establishment of selection criteria is readily influenced by personal preference, bias, and prejudice. The selection agent has both the legal and ethical obligation to be sure that the identified criteria actually address the issue of job performance.

In the health care industry, recruitment is rarely for the purpose of selecting one employee; more often there are several positions open and available at the same time. Consequently it can be efficient and effective for the selection committee to develop multiple criteria that are correlated with a position flowchart (see Fig. 2-4). This establishes a useful initial screening and routing procedure.

Once criteria are established, the process of selection is one of gathering, validating, interpreting, and passing judgment on candidate data relative to the criteria. The selector has four primary sources of information available: the application form, interview impressions, test results, and references from the past. Determining an applicant's fit with task requirements (i.e., aptitude, skill, experience) is most reliably done through examination of the application, references, and occupational skill testing. The fit with social and climatic aspects of the position (i.e., personal characteristics, physical appearance, leadership skills, career motivation, and social behavior and relationships) can best be judged through the interview and/or psychological testing.[11]

Each source of data provides its own types of information. Discussion of the relative merits of each is here presented in appropriate sequence for the selector: application, references, interview, testing.

Application. The application is the appropriate first step in validating essential requirements such as education, licensing, and specific experience. Additionally the application form provides information regarding general education, interests, past work experience (type, tenure, continuity, geography), and insight into the applicant's reasons for job searching. Subtly the applica-

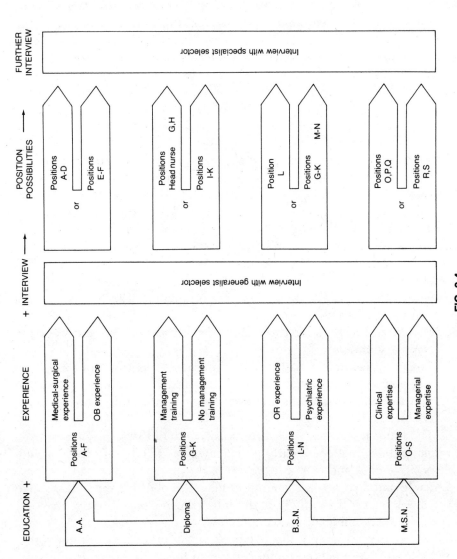

FIG. 2-4
Criterion-position flow chart. (Very loosely adapted from Seigel and Lane,[15] p. 86.)

tion bears witness to some personal attributes: neatness, writing skills, attention to detail, forthrightness. Application information may be utilized to reject applicants, to route applicants, or as a springboard for further dialogue.

References. References provide data regarding past employment. Information found in reference letters serves to support and verify data provided on the application. Past employment behavior is the best predictor of future employment behavior; the candidate's strengths and limitations as perceived by the past employer/supervisor are presented through references. Receipt of reference letters may result in rejection of an applicant either by identifying falsehoods or by describing behaviors that are contrary to the organization's needs or goals. It is worthwhile for the selector to exercise care not to overreact to negative aspects of a reference; they too can serve as a point of discussion.

Interview. The interview is the most time-consuming and therefore the most costly tool of selection. It is an interactive, interpersonal process identified as "the key predictor of the prospective employee's ability to fit into the organizational environment."[8] The interview seeks to establish personal and social skills, leadership desire and ability, and motivational level. The purpose is not to verify technical skills. The reliability of the interviewer's findings is inversely proportional to the number of criteria he or she is attempting to identify.

A good interview is a two-way learning interaction. Each party asks and answers questions. It serves as a forum for each to qualify the other to determine if continued negotiation/discussion is worthwhile. The interview process is fraught with many dangers:

1. The interviewer may be biased by information on the application form and behave in ways that activate the self-fulfilling prophecy.
2. The interviewer may be inexpert in communication skills, inept in generating discussion.
3. The interviewer may be overly sensitive to negative responses (especially those that come early in the interview) and be unresponsive to positive cues and responses.
4. Irrelevant factors (e.g., amount of makeup, obesity, apparel, sex, age) may detract sufficiently from the interviewer's objectivity to make his or her recommendations meaningless.
5. One party can modify the behavior of the other by avoiding certain topics or overreacting to other issues to the point of significantly distorting presentations of self.

Various styles of interviews have been described and developed. The most appropriate for interviewing licensed nursing personnel is a loosely structured interview utilizing open-ended questions. A rigid format will not provide enough of the appropriate kinds of information; stress interview techniques do not generate applicable data and would result in unnecessary feelings of discord. Adequate preparation is imperative in order to conduct a satisfactory interview. The interviewer should be thoroughly versed regarding the job, the employer, the terms of employment, and the requisite skills for satisfactory job performance.

The interviewing step in selection is a process of mutually qualifying the employee-organization match. It is fitting that at the close of the interview each person reassess and clarify his or her intent. The organization should state its case through the selector, and the applicant should indicate the extent of continued interest or disinterest. Summary statements are indicated and succeeding steps are discussed: What the next move will be, who will initiate future contact, and what the time parameters are for making a final decision.

Frequently and advisably, a second interviewer is utilized to confirm a decision to hire as well as to provide data for optimum placement. The ideal second interviewer is one who can more personally and intimately answer questions related to the task and the task environment. In order to facilitate sharing of interview impressions, a reaction sheet is useful. (Such an instrument is helpful to selectors because it clarifies and verbalizes their reactions, and it is more reliable than memory as the selection process continues.) A sample reaction sheet is shown in Fig. 2-5.

Testing. As a possible tool for the selector, testing is most effective when specific knowledge is indispensable and when particular technical skills are mandatory. Types, kinds, and numbers of preemployment tests are numerous. To provide optimum predictive ability, the test battery must be specifically chosen for the individual position. Psychological tests, if used at all, should be administered and interpreted by an expert. Testing that examines manual skills should be conducted in an appropriate setting and atmosphere. Preemployment physical examinations are almost universal. They are of course not reliable as predictors of future medical problems, but they do serve as a baseline indicator of health.

The process of selection is ideally a scientific one. Once criteria are established, candidates are reviewed and assessed who either meet the criteria and are hired, or who fall short of organization requirements and are not chosen. However, there are always circumstances that tend to modify science, such as urgency of need; ratio of applicants to the number of openings; rigidity or flexibility of criteria interpretation; and appeal, promises, and needs of candidates. The selector, as a human being, is involved. Many selection decisions are clear-cut; others require the selector to risk the organization's failing the potential employee or the candidate's failing the organization. It is this element of the task that provides the most challenge and potentially the greatest rewards.

Reaction sheet

Name of applicant _____

Date of interview _____

Position(s) being considered _____

_____

Overall impression _____

Social skills _____

Interpersonal skills _____

Leadership interest and skills _____

_____

Motivation _____

Verbal skills _____

Miscellaneous:

      Punctual _____

      Neat _____

      Thorough _____

      Other _____

Significant concerns _____

_____

_____

Discussed with applicant?   Yes _____   No _____

Specific strengths _____

_____

References on hand _____

Additional interview with whom? _____

Date _____

Applicant's significant concerns _____

_____

Next step _____

_____

Assignment _____

Date _____

Turnover data

          Date _____

          Reason _____

          _____

          _____

Next assignment _____

FIG. 2-5
Reaction sheet.

Conceptual framework

The selection portion of the employee entry process eventually boils down to either selection or rejection. En route, however, a series of choices is made by both the candidate and the organization that serves to ensure a mutually fulfilling relationship. Selection may be viewed as a series of eliminations, a process of evaluating the complements of requirements (see Fig. 2-6).

Skill requirements. Matching of skills occurs on the part of the applicant as a part of the recruitment phase. The potential employee has received enough positive responses to his or her inquiries to believe the position requires his or her skill levels. The organization typically determines skill fit through review of the application for education, experience, and licensure, routing or rejecting accordingly.

Reputation requirement. The assessment of reputation deals predominately with the past. The organization ascertains the candidate's reputation through references to past behavior from past employers in accordance with government regulations that apply. The interested applicant examines the organization for past policies, practices, and distinctions. It is significant that the past is predictive; it is also true that the new employee is immediately colored by the organization's past reputation and has the ability to modify the organization's repute.

Milieu requirement. Questions regarding future possibilities and present atmosphere must be answered. The organization presents its opportunities,

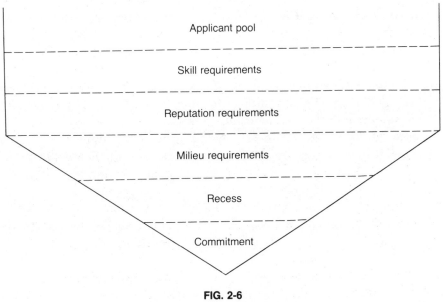

FIG. 2-6
Matching requirements.

reward methodologies, and potential parameters. The candidate shares his or her career goals, aspirations, and growth plans. The feeling tone of an organization has a powerful impact on one's development and growth potential. The organization is responsible for providing a growth-supporting milieu while supporting and reinforcing production.

Recess. It is possible occasionally to get carried away by the heat of the moment. Career moves have wide-ranging ramifications. Selecting employees has long-term implications. When selection is undertaken with an eye to retention, the choosing process becomes more serious. Economist Vetter describes an employee as "more than a current resource used in the production process. It has a long economic life which deserves the same planning attention given to other assets with long lives."[17]

Commitment. The last step in selection, commitment, solidifies the decision. Commitment statements could easily be, and often are, contracts; they are statements of terms, tasks, expectations, special understandings and privileges, contingencies, and time frames. A statement of rejection is a commitment too, an honest action based on valid data predicting an unsatisfactory alliance. The commitment interaction properly includes feedback for both candidate and organization, a mirroring of impressions to allow and facilitate mutual growth.

Critical issues and practical implications

Options. With the critical nursing shortage, persons assigned the task of selection see a limit to their options (i.e., either hire RNs or have a *very* good reason for not doing so). Clearly errors occur in selection: candidates are selected who fail (false positives); persons are not selected who would have succeeded (false negatives). The selector must decide which risk-reward route is most advantageous: risking organization resources through possible misfit and turnover, risking waste of human potential through too rigid rejection, risking personnel wrath through leaving the position open, risking little through selection of the perfect candidate.

Ethics. Stress placed on the selector can be tremendous. Expectations, hopes, and filling the role of savior/villain can tax one's standards. It is totally self-defeating, personally and organizationally, to misrepresent the truth or actually lie. Working in a third-choice area until an opening occurs in an optimum setting may become rapidly boring and counterproductive to satisfactory adjustment. It is ethically questionable and usually unsound to hire (select) candidates who have been at their present place of employment less than 1 year. (A further ethical note is relevant for the selector: that of honest reference data. A fair, factual presentation of past employee behavior is imperative to satisfactory selection. Such descriptions are not always available.)

Involvement. Involvement of the applicant's potential colleagues in the selection process increases the likelihood of success. Not only does this exchange provide necessary information for decision making; it also facilitates the transition and acceptance of the new employee. Heavy expenditure of staff time for interviewing interferes with productivity, so it is the task of the generalist selector to maintain a decision timetable. Staff members who are not routinely involved in decision making may find helping with selection difficult, implying the need for education and coaching.

Value. How much time is appropriate to spend on each candidate? Is there a formula? When is one wasting time? There are no neat answers to these questions but some may be inferred from other factors. A tenured employee is the most expensive investment an organization makes. An attitude that implies little consequence "if it doesn't work out" conveys a negative value to the candidate. It is often true that one gets back what one invests.

Openness. Selectors tend to like neat job descriptions and specially tailored candidates to fit into these positions. Because people tend not to fit into neat boxes and uniform molds, the selection process requires a considerable degree of creativity and flexibility to accommodate two sets of needs and even to foresee that accommodation is possible. Individual judgments and biases can handicap successful selection. It is imperative that persons involved in selection know their red flag areas and be on constant alert to their prejudices and areas of sensitivity.

Information versus privacy. Interviews can be stilted, uncomfortable, and superficial, or interactive, sharing, and explorative. The difference is not so much what is asked but how questions are asked, not so much the wording as the intent. In recent years, the regulations surrounding what one may or may not ask have grown remarkably. Consequently interviewers often feel tongue-tied and straitjacketed. It is worthwhile to (1) consult with the organization's legal counsel and (2) determine what you really want to know. "How old are you?" is inappropriate; "How long do you expect to work?" or "Are there physical limitations on what you can do?" are not. To ask "What religion are you?" is not acceptable, but the question "Will it bother you working with all nuns and priests?" is appropriate. Probing questions facilitate interchange. Nosiness is more repulsive (and illegal) in a professional than in a neighbor.

Assessment questions

For the organization:
1. What is your selection accuracy ratio?
2. How many appropriate candidates respond to your appeals?
3. At what stage are applicants most frequently lost?
4. How many applicants refuse your offers?
5. How open to creative selection is the organization?

6. Is the organization's community reputation consistent with the types of applicants you would select?
7. Have enough time and effort been devoted to establishing the correct criteria?
8. Are you demonstrating challenge, opportunity, and support?
9. Are your expectations realistic?
10. What is your reputation?
11. How much time elapses between application and decision?

For the selector:
1. What are your biases? How obvious are they? Do they get in the way?
2. What is your success ratio?
3. How are your interviewing skills?
4. Where do you make common mistakes?
5. What feedback have you gathered?
6. How have your failures affected the units? How have they affected you?
7. Do you always bring formal closure to all applications?
8. Which would you prefer, a false positive or a false negative?

For the staff member (unit):
1. Have you clearly defined your personnel needs?
2. Are you helpful in interviewing?
3. Have you been active in the selection process?
4. Do you prefer *anyone* or do you wait for a good fit? Have you communicated this desire to the selector?

PLACEMENT
Definition

Placement is the apportionment of talent. It is the act of commissioning a person to a position in a department where a supervisor or manager has accepted the individual. Appropriate assignment has a significant effect on both organization efficiency and individual satisfaction. Hampton[7] likens human behavior on the job to a large pair of scissors. One blade of the scissors involves the characteristics the person brings to the job; the other scissor blade includes the circumstances the job brings to the person. The task of placement is to fit these blades in ways that will allow the scissors to cut intricate, substantial, and quality patterns of job behaviors and performance.

Process

It would be convenient to rely on the "hope that the natural wishes and interests will push everyone to the place for which his [her] dispositions, talents, and psychophysical gifts prepare him [her]."[14] Assuring that people

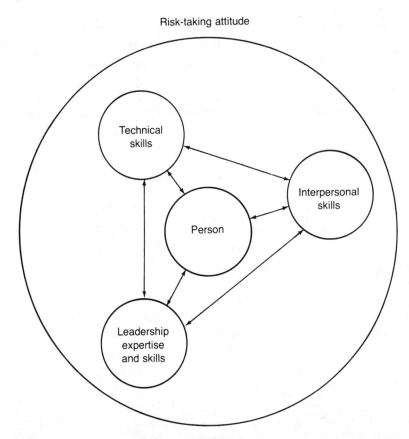

Risk-taking attitude

FIG. 2-7

The professional paradigm. (Copyrighted by Supportive Management/Educational Services (SMES), Ltd., 1979.)

find their place is, however, an active process. It implies intimate awareness and familiar knowledge of the organization, the individual, present personnel, and job requirements. It calls on placement personnel's skills of flexibility, creativity, risk taking, conflict resolution, confrontation, teaching, and assessment.

Knowledge and awareness of the organization can be gleaned from policy, plans, community relations, norms, human resource planning, management style, and the like. One beginning for organizational assessment may be in the assessment questions for the organization provided throughout this chapter. Responsibility for understanding nuances in job positions belongs to the placement person.

The individual candidate is a composite of skills, attributes, beliefs, and behaviors (see Fig. 2-7). The professional is first a *person:* a unique blend of interactions and experiences; someone in process, changing, acting and being acted on, capable of self-actualization, not a stagnant entity. The professional has and continues to develop *technical* skills, *interpersonal* skills, and *leadership* expertise and skills. Each set of skills interacts with the other and is influenced by the person's unique attributes. The professional takes action based on his or her *risk-taking* attitude and ability. Although it is impossible to actually divide the candidate into these distinct sections, it is true that placement frequently hinges on one element or skill set more than another (e.g., "He's a nice person, he'll get along on 6"; "She can read and interpret ECG printouts—put her in coronary care"; "She's quiet, she'll fit in with Ruth"; "He's gutsy, they need a risk taker in admissions").

Professional people need balance. It is important to use and develop all skill sets. Consequently, placing persons in positions that emphasize one component of themselves to the frustration of others does not bode well for job satisfaction or retention. Overused skill sets will hypertrophy, and underused skill sets will atrophy, causing distorted and discontented personnel.

Idiosyncrasies of present personnel are important factors to consider when placing new employees. There may be organization policies and procedures that apply (e.g., no sibling-sibling, husband-wife combinations on the same unit). Gossip, rumor, personal feelings, or personality clashes are not, however, pertinent to placement. Data that are relevant include management style, locus of control, degree of participative management, amount of interdisciplinary teamwork, unit practices, unit change quotient (i.e., disruptions such as remodeling or a new medication system), past turnover, adjustment problems, and requests for transfers. It is possible that in assessment of their practices, placement personnel discover leadership, personal, and personnel problems as well as growth and development needs. Responsible handling of these findings involves confrontation and planning for resolution, not modification of placement practices.

Assuming correct and thorough management of the previous steps in the entry process, the placement person has two sets of building blocks with which to build a wall of retention. On the one hand, the organization contributes its needs for creativity, leadership, stability, uniformity, time allocations, enthusiasm, people, credentials, innovation, experience, technical skills, spontaneity, harmony, and following. Individuals, on the other hand, present themselves with needs and desires for security, shift preference, money, leadership growth, advancement, stimulations, personal autonomy, personal involvement, challenge, routine, recognition, and variety. The measure of a retaining wall is in the match of the two sets of building blocks. Bricks for a strong wall fit as in Fig. 2-8, *A*. The probabilities of retention are markedly weakened by ill-fitting blocks or forced fusing of blocks (Fig. 2-8, *B*).

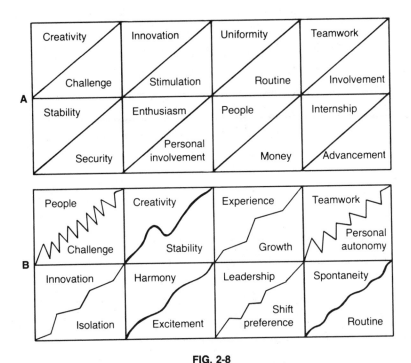

FIG. 2-8
A, The measure of a retaining wall is in the match of the pieces. **B,** The probabilities of retention are weakened by ill-fitting blocks or forced fusing of blocks.

Poor fitting is not only deleterious to an individual-organization relationship; it also jeopardizes the stability of the entire staff. The size of this retention risk is determined by the number, location, and size of the "weak bricks" (Fig. 2-9).

The consequences of initial placement are obvious. Faulty placement can result in sacrifices to organizational efficiency, threats to organizational integrity, frustration of personal and professional ambitions, and feelings of failure. Conversely, proper placement occasions growth, effectiveness, satisfaction, stability, and prosperity for both organization and individual. Ideal placement represents an integration of organization and individual goals, and is obvious through subsequent task accomplishment.

Understanding and knowledge of who should work where (the act of placement) are subject to change. People grow, gain more education, and change their desires, circumstances, feelings, needs, abilities, and relationships. Organizations react to changes in environment, community needs, competition, feedback, and profit-and-loss statements. They try new things; they discard antiquated methods and programs. As a result, the "best fit" changes. A method of answering the ongoing need for fluctuations, movement, and assessment will be examined in the context of conceptual framework.

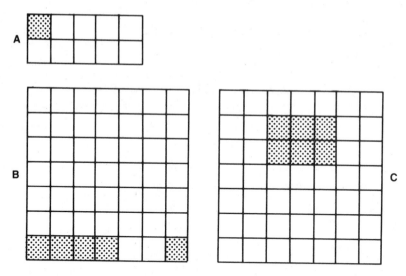

FIG. 2-9

A, One brick out of ten in peripheral (temporary) placement does not seriously endanger the wall. **B,** Another 10% may represent a critical threat to the entire staff if it constitutes the foundation of the organization (department), i.e., the director of nursing or supervisors. **C,** Faulty bricks in one place (one unit) can result in a hole in the wall with cracks that spread from that area.

Conceptual framework

It is said that a patient's discharge plan begins on the day of admission. Likewise an employee's career plan begins on the day of admission with the initial placement. The person most active in the employee's entry process has established a reflective, assessing relationship with the employee. Certainly the initial location has been identified. The placement individual is further responsible for teaching the candidate the system by describing the career charting procedure utilized by the organization. Organizations tend to be consistent in that entry processes are mirrored in transfer and promotion behaviors (e.g., luck versus planning, organization versus individual need, participative versus autocratic practices). Throughout this book, proactive, participative, growth-oriented practices have been advocated. The following placement and promotion conceptual framework incorporates these behaviors.

Each employee should have an individual professional growth chart (see Fig. 2-10). Where each intersection on the chart occurs, placement, learning goals, and estimated time to be spent in the position should be identified. Plateaus, transition periods, and turning points would then be identified and planned. Development of the growth chart should be a joint effort between employee and appropriate superordinate. The chart should represent both past experiences and future hopes; it should allow for both dreams and real-

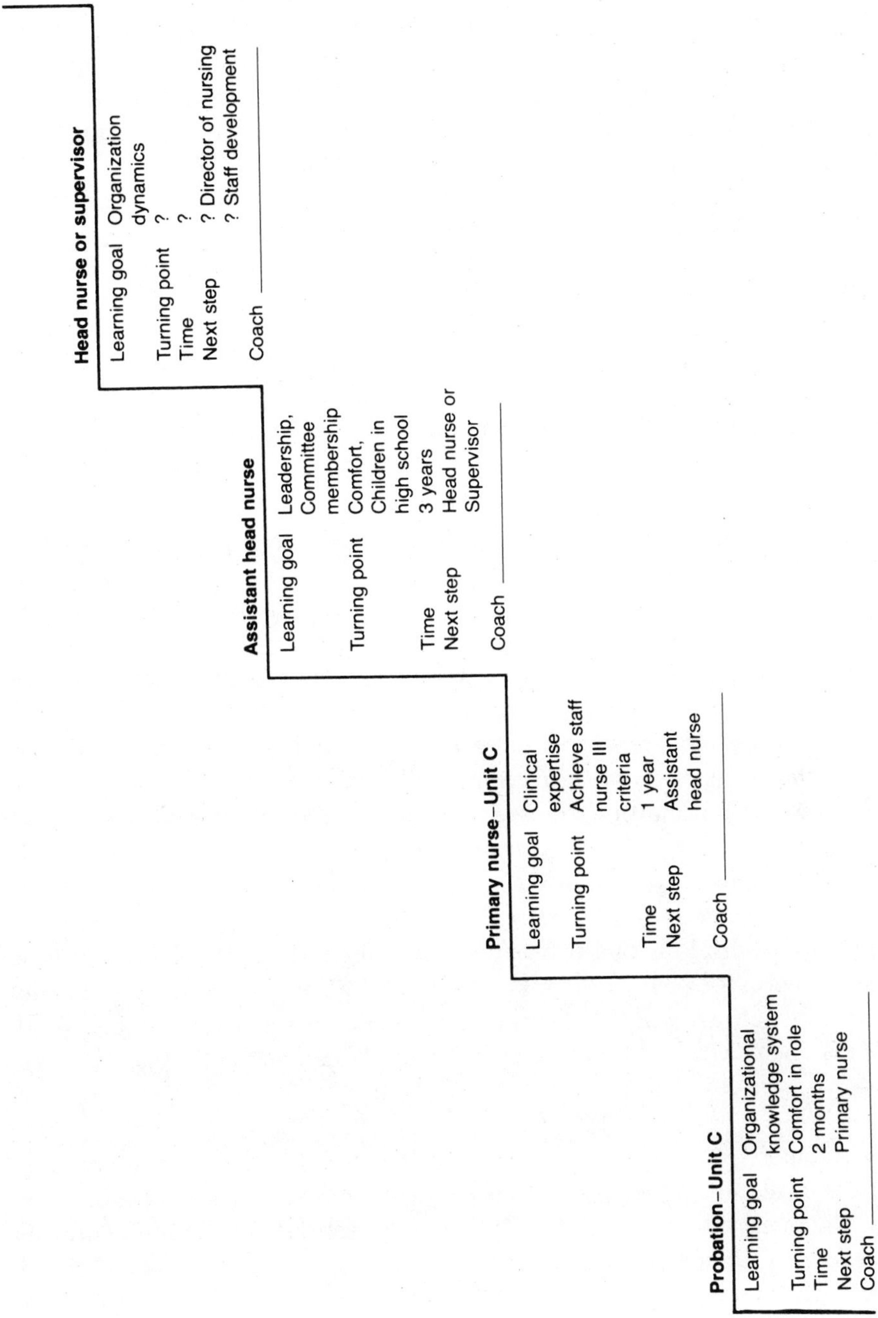

Head nurse or supervisor

Learning goal	Organization dynamics
Turning point	?
Time	?
Next step	? Director of nursing
	? Staff development
Coach	————

Assistant head nurse

Learning goal	Leadership, Committee membership
Turning point	Comfort, Children in high school
Time	3 years
Next step	Head nurse or Supervisor
Coach	————

Primary nurse—Unit C

Learning goal	Clinical expertise
Turning point	Achieve staff nurse III criteria
Time	1 year
Next step	Assistant head nurse
Coach	————

Probation—Unit C

Learning goal	Organizational knowledge system
Turning point	Comfort in role
Time	2 months
Next step	Primary nurse
Coach	————

FIG. 2-10
Professional growth chart.

ity. The superordinate functions include advising, supervising, educating, supporting, coaching, and recording.

Every placement along the growth chart is important. Building on the assumptions of the Morse and Lorsch contingency theory, it is understood that:

1. Along with a variety of needs, people bring to their work the basic need to achieve a sense of competence.
2. How this sense of competence is realized is individual and dependent on its interaction with the person's other needs.
3. Motivation to seek competence is most likely when organization task needs and individual needs fit.
4. Competency is an ongoing source of motivation; when one goal is reached, a higher one is established.

Individually charting and monitoring employees' growth has implications for both employee and organization. The individual knows his or her path and where to concentrate his or her efforts. There is a feeling of progression and of a competency-based motivation. Further, the coach ensures that the employee's progress is known and noted. This intimate current knowledge of its human resource inventory encourages organization effectiveness and efficiency. There is little room for the waste of human potential. The inventory appears as an actual file of employee information, listing (a) past experiences, (b) education, (c) pertinent skills, and (d) next targeted position. The system costs an organization coordination, planning, coaching, and education time; the results are an adequate supply of trained, groomed replacements, buoyed by system knowledge and organization loyalty.

A discussion of promotion, transfer, and placement is incomplete without at least reference to job posting. Job posting represents an organization's attempt to allow persons within the organization to apply for job changes. It is meritorious in its openness; accurate descriptions of vacancies are provided, self-nominations disallow bias from superordinates and allow a chance to skip levels. It also provides current employees the valuable opportunity to present themselves, to be assessed and interviewed, and to receive feedback. Job posting may be a worthwhile adjunct to other placement processes.

Critical issues and practical implications

Placement requires the melding of two composites, the individual and the organization, putting together many factors to generate the most complete picture. Given all the pieces of data, it seems appropriate to examine current practices as syndromes.

The squeaky wheel syndrome. This amalgamation of issues and events results in the placement of "best candidates" on those units with the most vocal representation. It stems from a desire not to have to listen to the same complaints of overwork, diminished patient care, and general maltreatment. It may or may not be coupled with the most critical organization need; it is simply the noisiest.

The urgency syndrome. The situation of urgency results from a blending of number and level of hierarchy requests for action. Threats to the integrity and usability of a unit contribute to this syndrome. Complaints or petitions from administrators, department heads, and clients will precipitate this behavior.

The safety-rut syndrome. The pattern of behaviors here referred to seeks clones of past successes. Replacing in kind is the norm. Nice, solid, noncontroversial candidates are valued. Creative assignments are unlikely; matching of personalities is more desirable than developing complementary alliances.

The ignorance syndrome. A mixture of excuses are characteristic of this behavior. "I wasn't told," "The file is out of date," "The information was not accurate," "There was no way of predicting. . . ." It usually covers inadequate preparation, insufficient time, poor communication, avoidance of conflict, unwillingness to confront, and/or fear of involvement. Much information from many sources is necessary to perform optimally. Lack of investment will be obvious.

The robot syndrome. The person exhibiting the robot syndrome denies responsibility and ability and functions as a supply clerk: "I gave them what they asked for." The special insights, creativity, and challenge needed for good placement are not exercised. Personal opinions, awareness, or involvement are absent.

The futility syndrome. The sad case represented here can result from burnout or apathy or gross ineptitude. "Flip a coin." "It really doesn't change anything." This mind set does not allow quality time expenditure. Believing it is all a matter of chance or that there will always be high turnover reduces the probability of effective assessment and placement.

The competence syndrome. A time- and value-laden approach, the competence syndrome does not allow rushed, precipitous decisions. It is long-term oriented, involving thorough exploration of the two sets of needs, and building lasting bricks and effective scissors.

Assessing one's typical syndrome may be advisable. Take the last 20 persons you were involved in placing. Identify which syndrome was most influential for each. As people tend to be creatures of habit, the first step in establishing new behavior is to identify present traits.

Assessment questions

For the organization:
1. What is your turnover rate?
2. How many personnel on exit interviews cite placement problems?

3. Which units or departments have chronic, "unsolvable" turnover?
4. What behaviors are valued as part of the entry process: Speed? Efficiency? Maximizing human potential?
5. Which policies affect placement? Are they current? Responsible? Appropriate?
6. How are new employees matched with positions? Is past experience or future goals emphasized? Which are more important: organization needs or individual preferences?
7. How are present staff educated and encouraged to assist in the adjustment of new members?
8. Are plans made and formalized for future placement? Transfer? Promotions?

For placement personnel:
1. Which syndrome best typifies your normal behavior?
2. What is your success ratio?
3. Do you inform new personnel about movement within the system?
4. What is your greatest skill? Your greatest liability?
5. Rate your knowledge of the organization.
6. Rate your knowledge of present job openings.
7. In your placement practices, are you risk taking? Cautious? Flexible? Rigid? Creative?
8. Have you identified trouble spots in the organization? Have you recommended (arranged for) help?

For the individual:
1. Have you plotted a career growth chart?
2. What skills are you developing or practicing?
3. Who is your present coach-mentor?
4. When will you be ready for a new assignment?
5. Does your supervisor know what role you want next? And when you will be ready?
6. Are you satisfied with your placement?
7. What skill sets would improve your unit? Have you shared these insights with anyone?

ORIENTATION
Definition

Orientation is the ability to locate oneself in one's environment with reference to time, place, and people; to ascertain one's true positions with respect to attitudes and judgments. The organization's formal orientation serves as a guide to facilitate new employees in orienting themselves in their new environment. The combination of time and activities that comprise *orien-*

tation is designed to provide sufficient information to enable the new employee to practice the professional skills he or she brought to the organization. "The organization must thereafter [following hiring] arrange circumstances to help its employees realize their potential for effective performance."[15] It is a time for investigating one's physical and emotional surroundings, one's colleagues and equipment, one's strengths and growth goals. It is a process of sharing expectations, defining relationships, and building communication patterns.

Process

The process of orientation is that of implementing a design, of carrying out a program. The person in charge may be likened to the director of a theatrical production. Responsibilities include providing the physical arrangements, identifying and procuring appropriate props, interpreting audience reactions, modifying timing, selecting and coaching actors, establishing and maintaining milieu. The simplicity of the task is, of course, complicated by audience participation. Nevertheless, the impact and significance of orientation rests in the design considerations, including goal, style, actors, topics, feedback, time, reaction, and conclusion.

The goal of orientation has become contaminated in recent years; the common present-day view of orientation is as a mixture of basic nursing education, remedial learning, and brainwashing with a fair dose of staff development thrown in. The goal of the orientation process is to *allow* employees to contribute, not to make them do things our way; to *set the stage* for satisfying job performance, not to create robots. It is inappropriate to design an orientation to augment abilities; that is the role of staff development. An employee is hired because he or she possesses certain needed skills. The purpose of the orientation phase of entry is to eliminate barriers to the successful practice of these skills.

The style of learning and teaching to be utilized is perhaps the most difficult decision to be made. That the learners are adults establishes certain parameters. The adult learner learns what has meaning and is necessary, is influenced by surroundings, learns best when he or she is committed, finds piecemeal learning irksome, learns best through use of more than one sense, needs to practice his or her learning, and progresses at his or her own pace. Acknowledging the commonalities of the adult learner, in addition, each individual has his or her own learning style. Each person relies more or less heavily on learning through concrete experience, reflective observation, abstract conceptualization, or active experimentation. Effective learning can occur by experimentation, analyzing and thinking, feeling, and/or reflecting.[10] Critical to useful orientation is the inclusion of all modes of learning, the flexibility to allow participants to learn in their own best way.

The actors identified for the part of teacher are significant on the basis of teaching style, expertise, perceptions of orientees, and place in the hierarchy. Including top managers in the orientation program provides an organization wide picture. It also assures their recognition by the new employees during day-to-day operations, thereby eliminating potential embarrassment from social ignorance. Utilizing the new employee's peers and colleagues for orientation establishes them as a team, including them in the responsibility for adaptation. The goal-related interaction fosters collaboration (positive interdependence) and diminishes the likelihood of competition (negative interdependence). The qualities required of a teacher of adults are those of a resource broker and helper who is able to structure learning, to diagnose learning needs, and to teach how to learn from human and material resources.[16]

Appropriate topics for inclusion in an orientation program are inexhaustible. Laws and accreditation guidelines offer some givens (e.g., fire, safety, and emergency procedures, patients' rights, job limitations). Traditions, expedience, and nicety also provide such offerings as physical surroundings, paydays, benefits, policies and procedures, schedulings, chain of command, peers. Efficiency suggests charting and recording procedures, supply locations, routines, assignments. Personal preference and organizational philosophies are reflected in the orientation topics. It is wise to include learner-generated topics throughout, to answer questions, and to discuss issues as they occur.

Learning is a lifelong activity; orientation is not. It is imperative to meet new employees' needs for security without threatening their ability to be self-directed. It is compulsory to familiarize them with organization methods without thwarting their creativity or undermining their education. Prompt introduction of new employees into the work force positively affects organization efficiency. Further, it significantly influences the quality of new interpersonal relationships. The longer one wears the label *novice,* the more difficult the transition to colleague and the slower the development of a sense of belonging and commitment. The greater the disruption of routine, the more likely are incidents of unfinished tasks, missed communication, and frustration. It is not necessary to teach new employees everything during orientation; it is mandatory for the long-term objective that they be taught how to learn and how to go on learning within the organization.

No learning situation is complete without feedback. A measure of the success of the program may be found in well-adjusted new employees, in job satisfaction, in satisfactory job performance, and in reduced turnover. Although these outcome criteria are important, gathering of data on the process of the program will allow continuous improvement as well. Quality grafting of new branches to the organization tree is significant to all employees. New members affect the quantity and quality of the teamwork as well as the reputation of the team. Consequently, openness to suggestions regarding orientation builds organization involvement, commitment, and morale.

The conclusion of orientation is identified by the goals that are described at the beginning of the program. It may be expressed in time, in proficiency levels, in task mastery. The task of orientation is complete when new employees feel comfortable to use their skills in the new setting. Other facets of orientation include recognition of one's place in the total organization, awareness of future possibilities, and knowledge of ongoing learning expectations and opportunities.

Conceptual framework

Throughout the orientation process, skills are taught, technologies are reviewed, certification may be updated; but the most significant occurrence is that of socialization. *Organizational socialization* "is the process by which an individual comes to appreciate the values, abilities, expected behaviors, and social knowledge essential for assuming an organizational role and for participating as an organization member."[12] The organization seeks through socialization to achieve high levels of individual performance with positive impact on group and organization output. Each organization is an ongoing social system that has "evolved a unique set of values, ideals, frictions, conflicts, friendships, coalitions."[5] It is the goal of orientation to enable the new person to enter this new system intelligently and to cope successfully.

Socialization includes an introduction to group norms, the values and modes of behavior that are respected. It is the price of admission. Group norms are established as "man's attempt at resolving a potentially explosive conflict of interest."[4] The two conflicting interests are (1) a desire for companionship and peer recognition, and (2) a human desire for autonomy and individuality. Group norms can be positive (supporting), negative (obstructing), or neutral (ineffectual). Orientation to group norms and organization norms is not meant to be indoctrination. Addition of new members can bring about attitudinal changes when they are allowed to impact on existing norms.

It is beyond the scope of this book to articulate a universal orientation program. The authors have attempted to raise relevant issues and ask cogent questions that must be answered by the individual organization. The tools, skills, and concerns explored in the section on program design in Chapter 5 may provide more specific help.

The function of orientation is to integrate individual and organizational needs while maintaining the integrity and self-confidence of the individual as well as the effectiveness and unity of the organization. As each individual is unique, so each organization is unique. The blending of these matchless entities without sacrificing either, and augmenting both of them, make up the

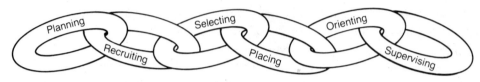

FIG. 2-11
Chain of entry into an organization.

special goal of orientation. The key assessment is one broad question (which may support its own series of questions): How successful are we in blending unique and new employees?

A CONCEPTUAL CONCLUSION

The process of entry into the organization has been described as a five-step activity. Five tasks are to be well executed to facilitate successful entry of new personnel. Five persons may be involved: (1) the planner forecasts human resource needs, (2) the recruiter supplies qualified applicants, (3) the selector chooses the best fit, (4) placement personnel assign employees where they can use their skills and develop new ones, and (5) the orientor demonstrates for the newcomer how to function in the new social setting. The accomplishment of each task and the investment of each person rests on the quality of work of each preceding task and the person doing it. Maintenance of an effective entry process is a team effort. Failure to behave professionally and thoroughly at any step jeopardizes the entire effort. This chain is truly as strong as its weakest link (Fig. 2-11).

The entire entry process is useless without adequate and skillful supervision. It does not occur in isolation from the rest of the organization. The persons involved in entry will continue to be involved with the employee, for gaining data on human resource needs, to ask assistance in recruiting, to facilitate transfers and promotions, to further educate. Therefore the means (entry steps) must be consonant with the ends (retention).

Introduction and first impressions are potent and long lasting. Investment of quality time in the entry process provides good long-run return. The effort expended to develop and maintain a first-class entry process is worthwhile *only if* the assumption is that one is hiring for retention and that individual employees are significant to the mission of the organization.

Frequently one of the five steps of entry constitutes a small section of a person's job description. Rarely are all five steps conducted by one person. This situation represents both strength and limitations for the process. A team approach is necessary (see section on team building in Chapter 3). Communication and coordination are imperative if applicants are not to be lost in the shuffle. Interdependence typically promotes awareness of one another and provides an excellent source of feedback, support, advice, expertise, insight, and help. The entry process team must interact; the ability to work well together requires effort and practice. Ongoing assessment and evaluation of this process and of the task are necessary in order to increase professionalism, develop sophistication, minimize mistakes, and maximize retention.

REFERENCES AND ADDITIONAL READINGS

1. Breaugh, J.A.: Relationships between recruiting sources and employee performance, absenteeism, and work attitudes, Acad. Mgmt. J. **24**(1):145, March 1981.
2. Coleman, B.: An integrated system for manpower planning, Business Horizons **12**(5):89-95, Oct. 1970.
3. Flippo, E.B.: Principles of personnel management, New York, 1976, McGraw-Hill Book Co.
4. Gibson, J.L., Ivancevich, J.M., and Donnelly, J.H., Jr.: Readings in organizations, Dallas, Texas, 1979, Business Publications, Inc.
5. Gibson, J.L., Ivancevich, J.M., and Donnelly, J.H., Jr.: Organizations: behavior, structure, process, ed. 4, Plano, Texas, 1982, Business Publications, Inc.
6. Groe, G.M.: Legitimizing human resource planning, Hum. Resource Plan. **3**(1): 11, 1980.
7. Hampton, D.R.: Selection and motivation, Hum. Resource Mgmt. **15**(2):22-29, 1976.
8. Jablin, F.: The selection interview: contingency theory and beyond, Hum. Resource Mgmt. **14**(1):2-9, 1975.
9. James, R.M.: Effective planning strategies, Hum. Resource Plan. **3**(1):1-10, 1980.
10. Kolb, D.A., Rubin, I.M., and McIntyre, J.M.: Organizational psychology: a book of readings, Englewood Cliffs, N.J., 1971, Prentice-Hall.
11. Lorsch, J.W., and Morse, J.J.: Organizations and their members: a contingency approach, New York, 1976, Harper & Row.
12. Louis, M.R.: Surprise and sense making: what newcomers experience in entering unfamiliar organizational settings, Admin. Sci. Quart. **24**(4):229-230, June 1980.
13. Mescon, M.H., Albert, M., and Khedouri, F.: Management, New York, 1981, Harper & Row.
14. Munsterberg, H.: Psychology and industrial efficiency, Easton, Pa., 1973, Hive Publishing.
15. Siegel, L., and Lane, I.M.: Personnel and organizational dynamics, Homewood, Ill., 1982, Richard D. Irwin, Inc.
16. Talking & Malcolm Knowles: the adult learner is a "less neglected species," Trng. Mag., pp. 16-20, Aug. 1977.
17. Temperley, S.R.: Personnel planning and occupational choice, London, 1974, George Allen & Unwin, Ltd.
18. Vroom, V.H., and Yetton, P.W.: Leadership and decision making, Pittsburgh, 1973, University of Pittsburgh Press. See also: Vroom, V.H.: A new look at managerial decision making, Organ. Dynam. **1**:66-80, 1973.
19. Wagner, B.: Bounties can't hide it: system swallows nurses, Am. Nurse **13**(7):5, July-Aug. 1981.

3

SUPERVISING FOR RETENTION

SUPERVISORY STYLE
  Beliefs
  Decision-making style
  Use of power
  Success
  Effect on retention, productivity, and job satisfaction
  Developing the best managerial style
SUPERVISORY AURA: TEAM BUILDING
  What is team building?
  What are the characteristics of a team builder?
SUPERVISING THROUGH SOCIALIZATION
  Components of socialization applicable to the supervisor
SUPERVISORY SKILLS
  Feedback
  Performance appraisal
  Delegation
  Decision making
  Problem solving
  Helping relationship skills
SUPERVISING TO RETAIN SELF
  Frustration
  Isolation
  Self-worth
  Facilitation toll
A CONCEPTUAL CONCLUSION

Supervisory relationships are aptly described as interdependent. The supervisor is charged with the responsibility of achieving production through others. The art of supervision is not simply a collection of activities, a prescribed set of behaviors; it is a process. Supervision is movement and change; it is alive, dynamic, and multidirectional; and it occurs over time. The supervisor is given charge of the organization's most costly investment, its employees. Therefore excellent supervision is the single most important factor in the success or failure of the organization.

What is expected of the supervisor has expanded since the overseer of biblical times and differs from that of captain of the chain gangs. The job description of the modern supervisor is multifaceted. It includes such behaviors as coordinating, directing, organizing, controlling, and staffing. It assumes communication, decision making, planning, and evaluating skills. It requires the ability to counsel, educate, motivate, represent, and develop staff. Much scholarly discussion has been devoted to differentiating among leading, managing, and supervising. For purposes of this text, however, it is assumed that the supervisor has an organizational vision (manager), the ability to inspire and motivate others to action (leader), and the assignment of facilitating and motivating the performance of others (supervisor).

Although state and federal laws, institutional regulations, and ethical and professional codes assign to all licensed nursing personnel the responsibility of monitoring and overseeing the care of patients, this chapter addresses the formalized role of supervisor. Insofar as he or she is directly responsible for activities of subordinates, the director of nursing or vice-president of nursing (executive manager), the supervisor or clinical care coordinator (middle manager), and head nurse or unit manager (first-line supervisor) are included in the definition.

The complexity of the hospital setting fosters a high degree of mutual reliance in interpersonal, intradepartmental, interdepartmental, and intraorganizational relationships. This interdependence, coordinated by the supervisor, may be either positive or negative. It may be characterized by cooperation and collaboration, or it may be based on competition and opposition. It can result in open sharing and assistance, or in conflict and rivalry. Supervisors have the monumental task of being responsive to the often conflicting needs of an individual, a unit, a department, the organization, the profession, and themselves.

SUPERVISORY STYLE
Beliefs

Variations in leadership styles have been traced to the supervisors' beliefs about people. Traditional managers believe that work is inherently distasteful to people, that few people are capable of work that requires creativity, self-direction, and/or self-control, and that pay is more significant to the worker than the nature of the job. Human relations managers believe that people want to feel useful, to feel important, to be integral to the organization, and to be recognized as individuals, and that these needs are more important in motivation than money. Human resource managers believe that people want to contribute to meaningful goals, want to help establish goals, and are capable of more creativity, self-control, and self-direction than is expected of them.[13]

McGregor[12] has provided additional supervisory labels based on beliefs. The theory X manager presumes the worker dislikes work, avoids work, has little ambition, desires security above all, prefers being directed, and requires external threat or coercion to put forth effort. The theory Y manager argues that work, both mental and physical, is natural and satisfying for human beings, and further believes that commitment to a goal will trigger self-directed behavior, which results in self-esteem and self-actualization.

The theory Z manager suggests that "productivity depends on trust . . . subtlety . . . and . . . intimacy,"[14] that involved workers are the key to increased productivity, and that productivity is a reflection on managerial organization.

Decision-making style

The manager's style may be categorized by his or her method of making decisions. An autocratic manager tends to make decisions alone with data presently available or with data gathered from subordinates. A consultative manager shares the problem with subordinates, either singly or in a group, to gather their opinions and inputs, but makes the decision independently. The group decision maker shares the problem and the decision with subordinates; willing to accept and implement any group-supported decision, the manager wields no power in the meetings but functions as chairperson-facilitator.

Participative management involves sharing of information and power with subordinates in both decision making and implementation. Its effective practice is based on the following assumptions:

1. Persons to be affected by plans and decisions should have a role in developing them.
2. Involvement results in investment of time, energy, and responsibility by the participants.
3. This involvement results in realistic goal setting.
4. The participative process is a method of working *toward* something (it is proactive).
5. Brainstorming stimulates creativity.
6. There are no preconceived solutions.
7. Alternative goals, views, and action plans are valuable.
8. The process involves orderly progression from idea formulation to action planning.

9. Participative planning presents an opportunity to practice collaboration and is a worthwhile experience in itself.

Use of power

The supervisor is granted certain powers by the organization: those of hiring, firing, transferring, promoting, developing, disciplining, praising, directing, and controlling, among others. Supervisory style is based on the exercise of these powers. Autocratic supervisors have power to impose their will on others and are not hesitant to do so. They will centralize power, rigidly structure subordinates' work, allowing them little or no latitude, and strictly enforce large bodies of rules that govern employee behavior. Autocrats are careful to oversee employees closely and to make thorough and frequent checks on behavior and output. Democratic managers elect to influence rather than control. They decentralize power, and develop and guide employees in their own decision making through openness, trust, and two-way communication. These managers attempt to broaden employees' perspectives by sharing information. Managers who abdicate all use of their power are called laissez faire. They exercise no influence or control over subordinates, allowing them essentially total freedom to establish their own goals and monitor their own progress.

Blake and Mouton[2] have coordinated managers' concern for task with their concern for people in the definition of five leadership styles, each of which exercises its hierarchical power in different ways:

1,1—The ostrich utilizes power through acquiescence, double-talk, and message passing.

1,9—The friend exercises power by smoothing, yielding, and suggesting.

9,1—The taskmaster uses power to master, dominate, and bring into line.

5,5—The fence sitter exerts power by seeking consent, compromising, and cajoling.

9,9—The executive uses power for consensus, confrontation, experimentation, and facilitation.

Tannenbaum and Schmidt[18] have examined the leader's use of power in terms of manager's and nonmanager's areas of freedom (see Fig. 3-1). According to this perspective, the more participative the manager's style, the greater the power of the nonmanager vis-à-vis decision making, and vice versa. Additionally, this model convincingly links power and influence with both manager and nonmanager work *behaviors*.

Success

Managers identified as high, medium, and low achievers have been studied and described.[7] Low-achieving managers are primarily interested in survival, avoid meaningful communications, quote policy and procedure manuals, do not involve subordinates in decision making, are concerned with job security, and distrust the intent and competence of their subordinates. Managers who achieve moderate success demonstrate a greater concern for production than for people, are preoccupied with their own ideas, listen only to superordinates, and are concerned with status and symbols of success. They distrust subordinates, do not involve them in decisions, and are pessi-

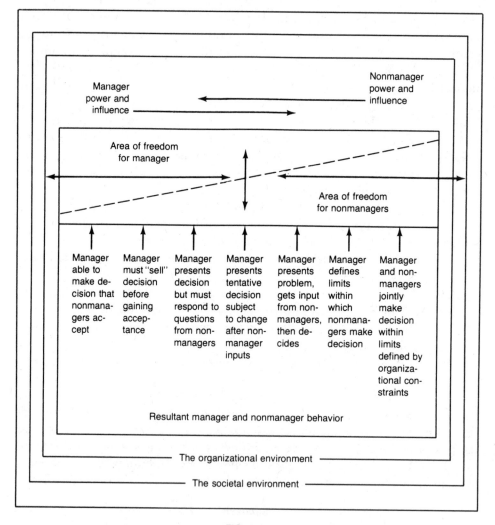

FIG. 3-1

How to choose a leadership pattern. From Tannenbaum, R., and Schmidt, W.: How to choose a leadership pattern, Harvard Business Review, May/June 1973. Copyright © 1973 by the President and Fellows of Harvard College. All rights reserved. Reprinted by permission.

mistic about people. Managers who earn the label of high achievers expect subordinates to do their best and believe their effort will be of high quality. Such managers are involved in providing employees with opportunities for self-fulfillment, rely heavily on the participatory ethic, and gather information from and share information with subordinates and superordinates alike. The high achiever has equal regard for production and people, believing organization goals and individual goals will be met concomitantly.

Effect on retention, productivity, and job satisfaction

Supervisory style can be and has been examined according to innumerable aspects. No attempt has been made here to present an exhaustive listing of supervisory styles. Rather, style has been described very broadly in order to focus on the impact of manager style on productivity, job satisfaction, and turnover. Additionally, although this text is not designed to diagnose manager style, it is advantageous for supervisors to identify their dominant, habitual style as part of examining the retention issue. Assessment of performance by self, peers, superordinates, and subordinates is an essential measure in addressing turnover.

The management philosophy of the organization tends to impact on one's preferred managerial style. Likewise, supervisory styles operate to modify an organization's style. The blending of these two belief systems into actual supervisory behaviors has profound effect on employees, their work, their job satisfaction, and their intention to stay.

- Believing employees dislike work results in mistrust, negative interdependence, diminished production, job dissatisfaction, and lack of motivation to stay.
- Believing employees require rigid and thorough structure results in uninvolved workers, missed tasks, uncooperative behavior, and frustrated workers who are very susceptible to turnover.
- Believing employees can be creative and desire involvement results in innovations, increased productivity, feelings of self-esteem, job satisfaction, commitment, and loyalty.
- Believing employees to be capable of self-direction and self-control leads to collaborative behavior, growth, experimentation, intrinsic motivation, and feelings of self-worth and self-actualization. These employees solve organization problems rather than seek new organizations.

Health care managers can learn from Japanese managers in the areas of power usage and decision making. Japan's average annual productivity growth from 1969 to 1979 was over 9%; the productivity growth of the United States for the past 5 years has been just over 1%. The average annual turnover rate in Japan is less than 5%; in the United States the rate is 25%. Franklin suggests "there are five qualities of Japanese management practices that are applicable to American businesses."[6]

1. "A longer-term view of business practice," including greater flexibility, regarding employees as investments, and training, transferring, promoting, and teaching them accordingly
2. "A partnership in the needs of firm and employee" involving mutual investment for the well-being of each in the long run
3. "Openness in organization structure and interactive communications," indicating liberalization of the hierarchical caste system with its incumbent distancing phenomenon; a discontinuance of gamesmanship and a building of honesty in interactions
4. "Sharing of organizational power. . . . People are a power source, and the job of management is neither to tend nor to tame but rather to release the power in people."
5. "An ongoing search for improving productivity" brought about by constant self-assessment on the part of the workers. Quality circles and workers' voluntary control groups function to critique practices and performance based on the belief that "work must be organized and equipped so that people are *able* to take responsibility for its quality."

Developing the best managerial style

The best managerial style in any situation results from the unique combination of three factors: the leader, the followers, and the situation. Individuals have personal styles made up of values, beliefs, confidences, inclinations, and feelings. Groups of would-be followers have their special characteristics compounded by group member makeup, history, goals, knowledge, experience, and individual needs. Situations vary by setting, severity, time parameters, and past practice. Health care managers are autocratic, democratic, and laissez faire, laid back and assertive, active and reactive, passive and insurgent, self-centered and other-directed, tolerant and insensitive, task master and friend. Followers in health care are trained and untrained, motivated and unmotivated, versatile and limited, aggressive, assertive, passive, and passive-aggressive. Health care involves crises, emergencies, watch-and-see situations, conservative and radical procedures, flexible and inflexible practices, personal and professional relationships, successes and failures, great joy and awesome grief. Identifying the peculiar mixture and evolving a practicable, appropriate supervisory style is the ongoing challenge and satisfaction of the health care supervisor.

Managing is a dynamic task, an unending stretching of self, a constant seeking and searching for new tools, and a devotion to growth and change. Persons seeking peaceful, status quo employment do not belong in management-supervision. The assignment of the supervisor is to bring about movement, to train the untrained, to motivate the unmotivated, and to energize, support, and provide growth opportunities for subordinates. The task is enormous. Mishandling of it results in stagnation, contamination, breakdown, waste, and turnover of the organization's most expensive resource: its people.

SUPERVISORY AURA: TEAM BUILDING

That quality or characteristic distinctive to a leader is the ability to build a team, the understanding and skill to generate collaboration, cohesion, and mutual reliance. Working cooperatively is a learned skill and not one that is fostered by our educational system. Competition has been emphasized; the individual is rewarded and responsible; students are taught not to share or ask for help, especially from one another; problem solving, from identification to taking action, is done singly.

Not every group is a potential team. "Teams are collections of people who must rely on group collaboration if each member is to experience the optimum of success and goal achievement."[4] Within organizations, work teams have the following characteristics:

1. Group has or will have a life together.
2. Group is accountable to a larger system.
3. Group members have varied authority, status, power, and accountability.
4. Group controls are often external to the group.

Effective groups have been described by several organizational development experts. Argyris[1] identifies three conditions that characterize effective organization units: (1) the ability to gather relevant data; (2) the ability to make sound, free, and informed decisions; and (3) the ability to implement those decisions with commitment.

Likert[10] lists the following, among others, as characteristics of an effective work group:

- Members are skilled in all the leader and member roles.
- The group has existed long enough to have developed relaxed working relationships.
- Group members are attracted to and loyal to the group.
- Group members have a high degree of trust and confidence in one another.
- Group members have helped shape the values and goals of the group and are satisfied with them.
- All interactions take place in a supportive atmosphere where communications are offered and received within a helpful orientation.
- The group is eager to help each member develop to his or her full potential.

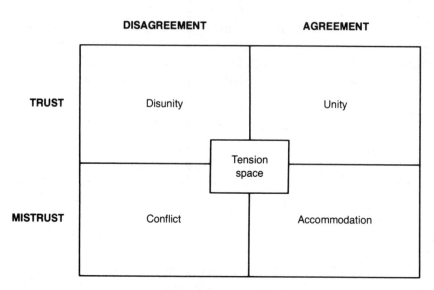

FIG. 3-2
Levels in group development.

- Goals are established that are challenging to each member without causing threat or anxiety of failure.
- Mutual help is common.
- Group members influence one another continuously.
- The superior in the group influences the tone and atmosphere of the group. "In the highly effective group, the leader adheres to those principles of leadership which create a supportive atmosphere in the group and a cooperative rather than a competitive relationship among its members."[10]

McGregor[12] defines an effective work team as one in which:
- The atmosphere is comfortable and informal.
- There is a lot of discussion.
- The task is well understood.
- The members listen to one another.
- There is disagreement.
- Decisions are reached by consensus.
- Criticism is common and constructive.
- Members express feelings as well as thoughts.
- Action is accomplished by clear and accepted assignment.
- Group power is shared.
- The group is self-conscious, taking time for process observation.

Groups can be examined by their level of trust-mistrust and their level of agreement-disagreement (see Fig. 3-2). Conflict will occur in groups with high levels of mistrust and disagreement. Groups characterized by agreement and mistrust will be accommodating. Trusting groups experiencing disagreement lack unity, whereas agreement and trust allow for united effort. Behavior within a group, whether trusting, mistrusting, agreeing, or disagreeing, will be modified by the feeling tone (noted by tension space in Fig. 3-2) of the situation.

In order for groups to perform satisfactorily, certain member behaviors are required. Specifically, two types of functions are necessary: those devoted to task accomplishment and those devoted to maintaining the group. Task functions include all behaviors directed to task completion: initiating, seeking, and giving information; clarifying, elaborating, summarizing, consensus testing, and recording. Maintenance functions are those interactions or actions devoted to keeping the group in good working order: harmonizing, gatekeeping, encouraging, compromising, including, and standard setting. There are also behaviors that interfere with group progress, for example, disrupting, blocking, attention seeking, dominating, and withdrawing. During the conduct of effective group or work team activities, the leadership functions of task and maintenance are shared and antigroup behaviors are confronted. The responsibilities for getting the job done as well as for keeping the team together are equally distributed. One's commitment to and valuing of the group is equally dependent on the quality of task and maintenance practices.

Groups and individual group members must resolve four key issues in their development. Each decides and from time to time redecides its stand on identity, goals and needs, power/control/influence, and intimacy. These items are presented in Table 3-1 in terms of questions that are answered by individuals and by groups in the interest of team functions.

The ability of the supervisor to build a team is significant because new teams need forming, established teams become less productive, functioning teams become dysfunctional, and barriers exist to collaborative behavior. Obstructions to cooperative endeavor stem from individual, group, and organizational sources. Individuals may be dependent or rebellious toward authority; they may experience difficulty in interpersonal relationships; and they may feel disequality among members and their influence in the team. Group members may have varying perceptions of the task or lack effective means of problem solving or decision making. The organization may offer financial or other rewards unfairly, present confusion regarding role expectations, or lack the means of solving intergroup conflicts.

Groups may be seen to be dysfunctional when they interfere with the achievement of organizational goals. Symptoms of this include:[4]

- Loss of production or unit output
- Increase of grievances or complaints among the staff
- Evidence of conflicts or hostility among staff members

TABLE 3-1

Individual and group concerns in four team issues

	Individual questions	Group questions
IDENTITY	Who am I in this group? How do I fit? Do I belong? Do I wish to belong? What behavior is acceptable here?	Who is welcome? How exclusive shall we be? How shall members be initiated? Are subgroups acceptable? What are our norms?
GOALS AND NEEDS	Does this group meet my needs? Are our goals the same? What does the group offer me? What do I give the group?	What is our purpose? How do we accomplish this? How do we judge our performance? Are personal feelings acceptable?
POWER, CONTROL, AND INFLUENCE	What influence do I have? What is my power source here? Am I controlled? Do I control?	How is the group to be led? How are decisions to be made? Who participates? What is the characteristic influence style? What kinds of power are accepted here?
INTIMACY	How close do I want to be? How personal can I be? How much can I disclose? How much can I trust?	Do we focus on task or process? Are personal issues acceptable? What is the atmosphere? How are confidences treated?

Source: Velthouse, B.A.: A workshop design, unpublished, 1982.

- Confusion about assignments, missed signals, and unclear relationships
- Decisions misunderstood or not carried through properly
- Apathy and general lack of interest or involvement of staff members
- Lack of initiation, imagination, innovation; routine actions taken for solving complex problems
- Ineffective staff meetings, low participation, minimally effective decisions
- Start-up of a new group that needs to develop quickly into a working team
- High dependency or negative reactions to the manager
- Complaints from users or customers about quality of service
- Continual unaccounted-for increases in costs

Established work teams may need renewal. This is especially true of groups demonstrating the Abilene paradox and groups that have become complacent. The Abilene paradox is the inability to manage agreement. It results in the group taking action in direct "contradiction to what they really want to do and, therefore, defeat the very purpose they are trying to achieve."[9] Symptoms of this include[4]:

1. Organization members feel pain, frustration, feelings of impotence, or sterility when trying to cope with the problem. In gross terms, there is a lot of apparent conflict.
2. Organization members agree privately, as individuals, as to the nature of the problem facing the organization.
3. Members also agree, privately, as individuals, to the steps required to cope with the problem.
4. There is a great deal of blaming of others for the conditions they are in.
5. People break into subgroups of trusted friends to share rumors, complaints, fantasies, or strategies relating to the problem or its solution.
6. In collective situations (group meetings, public memos, etc.) members fail to accurately communicate their desires and beliefs to others. In fact, they frequently communicate just the opposite.
7. On the basis of such invalid and inaccurate information, members make collective decisions that lead them to take actions contrary to what they personally and collectively want to do.
8. As a result of such counterproductive actions, members experience even greater anger, frustration, irritation, and dissatisfaction with the organization.
9. Members behave differently outside the organization. In other organizations (families, churches, other work units), they are happier, get along better with others, and perform more effectively.

Groups become stale. They drift along in a nice, safe routine with the same people doing the same tasks the same ways. Group members remark on organizational loyalty and devotion; productivity levels are unchanged from past years. Newcomers transfer out, risk-taking behavior is feared, and the group rewards solid, standard performance rather than creative or new ideas. Renewal and rebuilding allows for new satisfactions but is often resisted.

Often groups of "strangers" come together to work cooperatively. Being free of history, they do not find it necessary to break past habits; however, the group must establish a relationship, develop an accepting climate, and work out agreed-upon procedures. Committees, task forces, ad hoc committees, and project groups are a few examples of stranger groups common to the health care industry.

This section on supervisory aura has defined effective work teams; it has presented a number of organizational situations and symptoms that suggest team-building efforts. However, not every situation is appropriate for team building. As a supervisor, *do not build a team if*:

- You are uncomfortable sharing leadership and decision making with subordinates.
- The participants are not interdependent.

- The environment is highly stable.
- The hierarchy is rigid.
- The industry's technology is stable.
- Members of the management team are incompatible.
- Formal communication channels adequately convey necessary information.
- You are not dependent on subordinates for decisions on day-to-day operations.

A quick glance underlines the importance of team building in health care settings. The environment and technology are rapidly changing. Nurses and all health care actors are highly interdependent. Formal communication patterns are not adequate, and the bedside nurse carries the brunt of day-to-day operational decisions. Consequently, the major obstacles to team building can be identified as leader discomfort with shared decision making and/or incompatibility in the health care management team.

What is team building?

Team building is a series (not a one-shot event) of designed (not spur-of-the-moment) activities that focus on improving problem-solving abilities among team members. Team-building sessions include both "here and now" and "there and then" data, center around task and work issues allowing inter- and intrapersonal data as relevant to work, examine the group's relationship to the larger organization, and acknowledge feelings as being only part of reality. It is understood that the group comes together for more than just training and that significant work continues outside of the group.

"Process awareness is ... the essence of team building. When it understands and monitors its own process, a group is better able to accomplish its tasks and to utilize the talents of its group members."[15] Team building explores and examines the operations and emotions of the group's work; it concerns itself with what is happening between members while tasks are being accomplished. Appropriate topics for discussion include quantity, style, quality, and directionality of participation; influence styles; rivalry; hostility; decision-making procedures; task and maintenance functions; group atmosphere; membership; norms; and feelings. As group members gain skill in "processing" group behaviors, increasing openness and trust result, creativity and individuality become more valued, conflict is seen as energizing, and authentic feedback develops.

> The final aim of team building, then, is a more cohesive, mutual supportive, and trusting group that will have high expectations for task accomplishment and will, at the same time, respect individual differences in values, personalities, skills, and idiosyncratic behavior. Successful team building should nurture individual potential.[15]

Team building is carried out in day-to-day interactions by modeling and reinforcing the verbalization of process observations. A concerted, specialized effort, however, is required to change group behavior to impact significantly on its performance and character. Optimum team development programming begins with an off-site meeting for at least 2 days with everyone in attendance. It is imperative that expectations for such a meeting be realistic and shared. Although team-building efforts do not represent a cure-all, they do encourage dealing with difficult issues and increase the probability of participants getting feedback on their contributions to the group; and the impact will be felt beyond the involved group.

Five learning areas tend to result from effective team building. Group members gain:

1. Insight into themselves
2. Understanding of others and awareness of one's impact on them
3. Better understanding of group processes and increased skill in achieving group effectiveness
4. Increased recognition of the characteristics of the larger social system
5. Greater awareness of the dynamics of change

What are the characteristics of a team builder?

Most important are the facilitator's beliefs and values. Belief in the integrity and abilities of people is fundamental. Valuing of self-expression, creativity, authenticity, self-control, and self-direction for self and others is imperative. Knowledge and experience are necessary for success. Understanding of human functioning, knowledge of group interaction and dynamics, and theoretical comprehension of specific group facilitation styles are required. Experience as a group member and facilitator trainee are essential. Familiarity and flexibility with tools of the trade generate greater comfort and breadth of the experience for participants. Simulation, self-assessment instruments, counseling, consciousness raising, values clarification, sensory awareness, and biofeedback and relaxation methodologies may all be required.

> The possibility that a work unit could exhibit public equanimity, private turmoil, and perform ineffectively is one compelling reason for work groups to hold periodic team review and development sessions. . . . Another reason is that the organization might be able to do something constructive about the problem, even though the skills required for success in such a session may not be easy or comfortable to learn.[4]

On pp. 86-92 is a series of assessment instruments that will help a group that wants to examine itself to establish need for team building, renewal, renovation, and/or support. For additional assessment instruments, see William Dyer's *Team Building: Issues and Alternatives.*[4]

Text continued on p. 93.

SOME DIMENSIONS OF GROUP EFFECTIVENESS

Directions: Place a check mark along each scale, showing about where you would rate this group at this time.

A. Task functions

1. How clear are the goals in this group?

0	1	2	3	4	5	6	7
Utter confusion		Hidden agendas		Average	Fairly clear now		Clear focus shared by all

2. How strongly involved do we feel in what this group is doing?

0	1	2	3	4	5	6	7
Couldn't care less	Not much interest		Average		Interested		Deeply involved and concerned

3. How well do we diagnose our group problems?

0	1	2	3	4	5	6	7
Avoid, try to disregard	Slight attention		Average		Considerable attention		Face frankly; analyze with care; successful diagnosis

4. How appropriate are our group norms and procedures for our group goals?

0	1	2	3	4	5	6	7
Defeating our purpose	Not much help		Average		Often fitting; useful		The best possible means to our ends

5. How well do we integrate contributions from various members?

0	1	2	3	4	5	6	7
Each goes it alone; has his or her say, disregards others No summary or integration		Slight attention to others' ideas		Average	Considerable attention to using ideas of others		Each speaks; builds directly on contributions from others; relates; ties together

6. How do we usually make decisions?

0	1	2	3	4	5	6	7
We don't. Plop.	Self-authorized	Hand clasp	Minority	Majority	False consensus (silence as consent)	Forced consensus	True consensus

7. How do we mobilize the potential resources and creativity of our members for accomplishing our goals?

0	1	2	3	4	5	6	7
No one contributes freely; resources are unused		Only a few contribute		Average	Most members contribute a great deal		Everyone contributes fully and creatively

B. Maintenance functions

8. How much do members enjoy working with the others in this group?

0	1	2	3	4	5	6	7
All hate it; ready to quit		Discontented	Average Some do not care; some displeased		Rather pleased; some enjoyment		All love it; real joy; strong cohesion

9. How much encouragement, support, and appreciation do we give to one another as we work?

0	1	2	3	4	5	6	7
None	Seldom give support		Average Some appreciated; some ignored; some criticized		Often give support		Abundant for every member even when we disagree

10. How freely are our personal and group feelings (both affectionate and hostile) expressed?

0	1	2	3	4	5	6	7
No feelings expressed; all work oriented		Seldom express feelings, only negative ones or only positive ones	Average Expressed when unusually strong		Often express feelings both positive and negative		Both personal and shared feelings expressed by all

Continued.

SOME DIMENSIONS OF GROUP EFFECTIVENESS—cont'd

B. Maintenance functions—cont'd

11. How constructively are we able to use disagreements and conflicts in this group?

0	1	2	3	4	5	6	7
Avoid or repress them; or, so bad they threaten to break up the group		Seldom examine conflicts		Average Smooth them over; change the subject; occasional constructive exploration	Often explore conflicts		Welcome them, explore them, find them most valuable

12. How sensitive and responsive are we to the feelings of others that are not being overtly expressed?

0	1	2	3	4	5	6	7
Blind, insensitive, unconcerned, inert, ruthless		Seldom notice them	Average Only occasional responses to such feelings		Often respond to them		Fully aware, very sensitive, very responsive

13. How frequently do we give nonevaluative feedback that other members can connect directly with specific behaviors?

0	1	2	3	4	5	6	7
Never give any; or give only "right" and "wrong" judgments		Rather seldom	Average		Fairly often		Very frequently given and well received

14. How many members are experiencing new understanding of themselves, seeing new facets of others, experiencing changes in outlook and perspective, have a sense of growth and self-realization?

0	1	2	3	4	5	6	7
None	A few		About half		Most		All

TEAM-BUILDING CHECKLIST

I. Problem identification: To what extent is there evidence of the following problems in your work unit?

	Low evidence		Some evidence		High evidence
1. Loss of production or work unit output	1	2	3	4	5
2. Grievances or complaints within the work unit	1	2	3	4	5
3. Conflicts or hostility between unit members	1	2	3	4	5
4. Confusion about assignments or unclear relationships between people	1	2	3	4	5
5. Lack of clear goals, or low commitment to goals	1	2	3	4	5
6. Apathy or general lack of interest or involvement of unit members	1	2	3	4	5
7. Lack of innovation, risk taking, imagination, or taking initiative	1	2	3	4	5
8. Ineffective staff meetings	1	2	3	4	5
9. Problems in working with the boss	1	2	3	4	5
10. Poor communications: people afraid to speak up, not listening to each other, or not talking together	1	2	3	4	5
11. Lack of trust between boss and member or between members	1	2	3	4	5
12. Decisions made that people do not understand or agree with	1	2	3	4	5
13. People feeling that good work is not recognized or rewarded	1	2	3	4	5
14. People not encouraged to work together	1	2	3	4	5

Scoring: Add up the score for the 14 items. If your score is between 14 and 28, there is little evidence your unit needs team building. If your score is between 29 and 42, there is some evidence, but no immediate pressure, unless two or three items are very high. If your score is between 43 and 56, you should seriously think about planning the team-building program. If your score is over 56, then building should be a top-priority item for your work unit.

II. Are you (or your manager) prepared to start a team-building program? Consider the following statements. To what extent do they apply to you or your department?

	Low	Medium			High
1. You are comfortable in sharing organizational leadership and decision making with subordinates and prefer to work in a participative atmosphere.	1	2	3	4	5
2. You see a high degree of interdependence as necessary among functions and workers in order to achieve your goals.	1	2	3	4	5
3. The external environment is highly variable and/or changing rapidly and you need the best thinking of all your staff to plan against these conditions.	1	2	3	4	5
4. You feel you need the input of your staff to plan major changes or develop new operating policies and procedures.	1	2	3	4	5
5. You feel that broad consultation among your people as a group in goals, decisions, and problems is necessary on a continuing basis.	1	2	3	4	5
6. Members of your management team are (or can become) compatible with each other and are able to create a collaborative rather than a competitive environment.	1	2	3	4	5

From Dyer, W.G.: Team building, issues and alternatives, Reading, Mass., 1978, Addison-Wesley Publishing Co., pp. 36-40. Reprinted with permission.

Continued.

TEAM-BUILDING CHECKLIST—cont'd

	Low	Medium	High

7. Members of your team are located close enough to meet together as needed.   1   2   3   4   5

8. You feel you need to rely on the ability and willingness of subordinates to resolve critical operating problems directly and in the best interest of the company or organization.   1   2   3   4   5

9. Formal communication channels are not sufficient for the timely exchange of essential information, views, and decisions among your team members.   1   2   3   4   5

10. Organization adaptation requires the use of such devices as project management, task forces, and/or ad hoc problem-solving groups to augment conventional organization structure.   1   2   3   4   5

11. You feel it is important to surface and deal with critical, albeit sensitive, issues that exist in your team.   1   2   3   4   5

12. You are prepared to look at your own role and performance with your team.   1   2   3   4   5

13. You feel there are operating or interpersonal problems that have remained unsolved too long and need the input from all group members.   1   2   3   4   5

14. You need an opportunity to meet with your people, and to set goals and develop commitment to these goals.   1   2   3   4   5

Scoring: If your total score is between 50 and 70, you are probably ready to go ahead with the team-building program. If your score is between 35 and 49, you should probably talk the situation over with your team and others to see what would need to be done to get ready for team building. If your score is between 14 and 34, you are probably not prepared at the present time to start team building.

III. Should you use an outside consultant to help in team building? (Circle appropriate response.)

1. Does the manager feel comfortable in trying out something new and different with the staff?   Yes   No   ?

2. Is the staff used to spending time in an outside location working on different issues of concern to the work unit?   Yes   No   ?

3. Will group members speak up and give honest data?   Yes   No   ?

4. Does your group generally work well together without a lot of conflict or apathy?   Yes   No   ?

5. Are you reasonably sure that the boss is not a major source of difficulty?   Yes   No   ?

6. Is there a high commitment by the boss and unit members to achieve more effective team functioning?   Yes   No   ?

7. Is the personal style of the boss and his or her management philosophy consistent with a team approach?   Yes   No   ?

8. Do you feel you know enough about team building to begin a program without help?   Yes   No   ?

9. Would your staff feel confident enough to begin a team-building program without outside help?   Yes   No   ?

Scoring: If you have circled six or more "yes" responses, you probably do not need an outside consultant. If you have four or more "no" responses, you probably do need a consultant. If you have a mixture of yes, no, and ? responses, you should probably invite a consultant to talk over the situation and make a joint decision.[4]

PROBLEM-SOLVING OR GROUP-BLOCKING DIAGNOSIS FORM*

Which behaviors more typify your team, problem solving or group blocking? Check all behaviors which characterize your group's activities.

Problem-solving behaviors	Blocking behaviors
____ Clarifying	
____ Summarizing	____ Ambiguity
____ Testing	____ Overgenerality
____ Informing	____ Too early evaluation
____ Giving ideas	____ Status threatening
____ Reality testing	____ Inexperience
____ Harmonizing	____ Straw voting
____ Compromising	____ Polarizing
____ Consensus testing	____ Failure to try
____ Feasibility testing	____ Failure to assign responsibility
____ Initiating	____ Lack of involvement
____ Taking action	____ Failure to follow through
____ Pooling resources	____ Lack of commitment
____ Process observing	____ Poor time utilization
____ Checking	____ Failure to take responsibility
____ TOTAL	____ TOTAL

Whenever blocking behaviors outnumber problem-solving behaviors, team building is needed. Also, a score of less than 8 on problem solving and 5 or more in blocking suggests team-building activities should be initiated.

*Copyright, Betty A. Velthouse, 1982.

A TEAM-ASSESSMENT FORM FOR THE SUPERVISOR*

The following questions may advantageously be asked of team members. Ascertaining their impressions verifies the supervisor's observations and sharpens members' process skills and feelings of group responsibility. Although anonymity may be facilitative early in group assessment, these questions can also serve as a team-building activity when discussed jointly.

What is the feeling tone of the work group?

Are members equally committed to group goals?

Do members take initiative in addressing group issues?

Do members "own" their thoughts, feelings, reactions (use "I" statements)?

Do members cooperate?

*Copyright, Betty A. Velthouse, 1982.

Continued.

A TEAM-ASSESSMENT FORM FOR THE SUPERVISOR—cont'd

How do members interact?
- Through self-disclosure?

- By expressing feelings?

- By supporting one another?

- By confronting one another?

What is the trust level?

Are members authentic in communication? Are there double messages?

What leadership functions are carried out and by whom?

Is there anxiety?

What mechanisms are used to escape problem solving? (Analysis, interpretation, pairing, withdrawal, personal aggression, fault-finding)

- How often does it occur?

What is needed to improve the quality of the group?

SUPERVISING THROUGH SOCIALIZATION

Organizational socialization is the process of learning the ropes, the process of being indoctrinated and trained, the process of being taught what is important in an organization or some subunit thereof. The concept refers to the process by which a new member learns the value system, the norms, and the required behavior patterns of the society, organization, or group which s/he is entering. This learning adaptation is the price of membership. "The speed and effectiveness of socialization determine employee loyalty, commitment, productivity, and turnover. The basic stability and effectiveness of organizations therefore depends upon their ability to socialize new members."[17]

The issue of socialization is discussed here rather than as a portion of orientation because of its pervasive nature, its impact on turnover, and the responsibility of the supervisor relative to it. That socialization is necessary for organization survival has been acknowledged. This socialization includes the goals of the organization, the means of goal accomplishment, the role responsibilities assigned each member, required behavior patterns, and those regulations that protect the identity and integrity of the organization. Sadly, not all of socialization is constructive. Portions of the process include destruction, demoralization, intimidation, and restriction. Old behavior patterns are deemed unsound, past experience is undervalued, commitment and integrity are questioned, education and knowledge are inconsequential or ill-fitting. Adsorption into an organization is a course of upheaval.

Three reactions to the socialization process are common: "rebellion, creative individualism, and conformity."[17] Rebellious employees reject all values, norms, expectations, and behaviors. They either leave the organization (turnover) or create unrest. Conforming individuals accept all norms, values, beliefs, and practices; they cease all creativity and mimic their co-workers. Both of these reactions represent organization failures; neither will contribute to the vitality or growth of the organization; one is bent on destruction, one on sterility. The creative individual accepts only those norms and values that are essential for job and organization effectiveness. This person retains individuality, objectivity, and creativity while joining in to fulfill the organization mission.

Socialization is typically discussed as it relates to newcomers, that is, persons new to a family, new to an institution, new to a culture. However, socialization is an ongoing process; behaviors are accepted and reinforced and we are resocialized with more deeply entrenched beliefs and values. Consider this in relation to a nursing unit with high turnover. Certain values and norms are counterproductive to the organization's goals, yet unit members are being socialized and resocialized to conform to these models. Supervisors cannot be held entirely responsible for socialization as it occurs in areas under their direction. However, it is legitimate to expect supervisors to be aware of the process of socialization (both strengths and limitations) as it occurs on units assigned to them and to hold them accountable for the appropriateness of the norms and values espoused by the personnel on those units.

Socialization that results in group and organization membership is a source of both security and insecurity for the individual; it may provide satisfaction or frustration. Group membership demands some degree of conformity in behavior, attitude, beliefs, and values; it tends to determine self-esteem, it requires certain interpersonal skills, and it is almost universal in organizational life. Persons tend to be members of more than one group at a time, which can cause conflict. Groups develop a personality of their own. Groups can become sick and they can change; thus groups require regular self-assessment and performance appraisal.

> The essence of management is to understand the forces acting in a situation and to gain control over them. It is high time that some of our managerial knowledge and skill be focused on those forces in the organizational environment which derive from the fact that organizations are social systems who do socialize their new members. If we do not learn to analyze and control the forces of organizational socialization, we are abdicating our primary managerial responsibilities.[17]

Although supervisors cannot assess, control, or change a group alone, they can facilitate group self-examination. It is recommended that supervisors in conjunction with their work group assess components of their socialization process in light of (1) its role in retention-turnover, (2) its appropriateness, (3) its acceptability to all members, (4) its impact on productivity, and (5) potential changes.

Components of socialization applicable to the supervisor

Values. Values are personal ideas, abstract beliefs that describe or represent one's definition of the ideal. People value certain behaviors, certain feelings, certain attitudes. Values affect what one does, how one perceives another, how one prioritizes tasks, and how one behaves toward another. Persons with values similar to one's own are more well liked than those with contrasting beliefs. However, a work group with great homogeneity of values tends to become cohesive to the point of isolationism, rigid to the point of defensiveness; this results in reduced productivity, interdepartmental conflict, and a highly selective clientele. Work groups that contain a variety of values along with a wide range of value acceptance will be able to serve a broader audience, provide more varied services, accept new members, and try new things.

Norms. Norms are standards that regulate *behavior*. They do not relate to thoughts or feelings. They develop gradually, may be explicitly stated or implicitly understood, or may operate completely below the group's level of

TABLE 3-2

Behaviors and norms

Categories of behavior		
Individual	**Interpersonal**	**Norms**
Experimenting	Help others to experiment	Trust
Openness	Help others to be open	Concern
Owning	Help others to own	Individuality
Zero line		
Not owning	Not help others to own	Conformity
Not open	Not help others to be open	Antagonism
Rejecting experimentation	Not help others to experiment	Mistrust

From Argyris, C.: The incompleteness of social psychological theory: examples from small group, cognitive consistency, and attribution research, New Haven, Conn., 1970, Department of Administrative Sciences, Yale University, p. 895.
NOTE: Categories above the zero line are hypothesized to facilitate interpersonal relationships, those below the line to inhibit interpersonal relationships. Categories positioned closest to zero line are easiest to perform and those farthest away the most difficult.

awareness. Table 3-2 identifies certain norms with their resultant behaviors.

Conformity versus creativity. Too much conformity leads to stagnation; too much creativity results in chaos. Employees are hired to both create and conform. The entry process informs candidates that the organization values them for their insight, ability, and education; the socialization process clearly outlines *how things are done here.* Optimum balance between creativity and conformity is a function of group members, organizational objectives, and supervisor flexibility. It is important to recognize that individual risk taking is dependent on the person's sense of security in the group as well as the belief in the supportiveness of the group. Further, the supervisor's appetite for growth and change, his or her aptitude at facilitating and encouraging creativity, will either generate or squelch imagination.

Interdependence. Interdependence, the fact of mutual reliance, may be interpreted as either collaboration or competition (see Fig. 3-3). The degree of harmony (positive interdependence) within a group is a function of the degree to which members perceive a common goal that is mutually compelling and unreachable unless each member exerts an effort. Healthy conflict is a natural occurrence wherever creative, intelligent people work together. However, this is not the type of conflict referred to in the figure; healthy conflict is resolved allowing for expansion of ideas; unhealthy conflict is sustained for its own sake.

Coaching. Coaching involves observing, analyzing, commenting, and offering suggestions on how one can improve performance. Coaching is not designed for staff development but for adequacy in performance. It is a su-

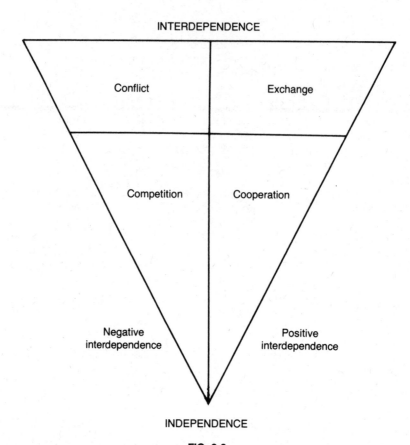

FIG. 3-3

Interdependence possibilities. From Thurkettle, M.A., and Jones, S.L.: Conflict as a systems process: theory and management, J. Nurs. Admin., Jan. 1978.

pervisory responsibility; it is performed by supervisors, subordinates, and peers as well. Coaching is most beneficial when it is carried out by a good role model, is built on strengths, broadens one's perspective, and is accompanied by specific examples. Coaching is an important supervisory skill; its potential danger to retention lies in its overuse. It is possible to fall into a teaching-coaching relationship that stifles self-direction and disallows differences.

Relationships. Employees are very susceptible to the subtle pressures of propriety that prescribe relationships. Such pressures involve both norms and procedures; they dictate who talks to the doctor and how the chain of command operates. Nuances tell employees whom they should talk to about what, whether it is OK to problem solve with another department or to let the supervisor do it. Often the socialization issues regarding relationships are based on unvalidated perceptions of another's sense of security. Too often they interfere with productivity.

Self-fulfilling prophecy. Neither a norm nor a value, the concept of the self-fulfilling prophecy is a pervasive component of socialization and turnover. The concept includes a wide range of beliefs and behaviors that have consequences for socialization. Self-fulfilling prophecy simply stated is the tendency for things to turn out as one predicts. It is important to note that this is not magical; rather, in subtle, often unconscious ways, one "helps" things to turn out this way. The significance of the concept for socialization is this: If we, or the work group, expect a person to fail, that individual will be "helped" to fail. If we expect turnover, resistance, and personality clashes, they will occur. If the expectation is for long-time employment, creativity, flexibility, cooperation, and effort, these behaviors are likely to be forthcoming.

SUPERVISORY SKILLS

A comprehensive listing of supervisory skills is beyond the scope of this book. Instead we have chosen to address those skills most relevant to retention: feedback, performance appraisal, delegation, decision making, problem solving, and helping relationship skills.

Feedback

Feedback is a way of giving help. It serves the function of being a mirror to the individual, an unbiased description of his or her behavior. Consequently, feedback is descriptive rather than evaluative, specific rather than general, focused on behavior rather than the individual; and it involves shared information rather than advice. Helpful feedback is that which is directed toward behavior the receiver can alter. It is well timed, it involves the amount of information the receiver can use, and it is checked for understanding. Feedback avoids such words as good, bad, always, never, you should, you might, because; it avoids emotion-laden words and is succinct, specific, and honest. Attention is paid to the results of giving feedback.

As feedback is most likely to be valued when it is solicited, it is important for the supervisor to encourage and to teach subordinates how to ask for feedback. Perhaps the most significant issue here is trust. Believing the supervisor to be honest, authentic, valuing growth, and desiring to help will enable subordinates to seek that mirror. Availability, openness, and modeling (asking others for feedback) are other qualities that make feedback a used and useful tool.

Performance appraisal

The performance appraisal process is directed toward growth. It is too often contaminated with disciplinary issues. Discipline is directed toward behavior change for the good of the *organization*. Performance appraisals also tend to promote change, but they are self-directed and exist for *personal* and *professional* growth. Performance appraisal involves a process, a form, and a meeting. The performance appraisal process is well depicted in the Colby and Wallace[3] paradigm (see Fig. 3-4). The annual meeting is only a part of the interaction.

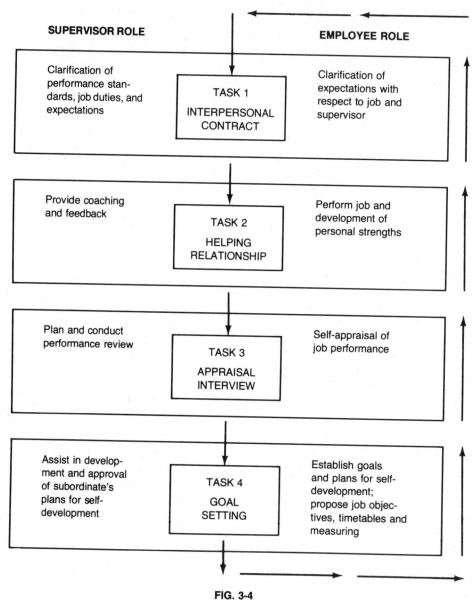

FIG. 3-4

Supervisor and employee roles in performance appraisal. From Colby, J.D., and Wallace, R.L.: Performance appraisal: help or hindrance to employee productivity? Personnel Administrator **20**:37, Oct. 1975.

ASSESSING PERFORMANCE APPRAISAL SESSIONS:
A CHECKLIST FOR MANAGERS*

KEY: (1) No; (2) mostly no; (3) neutral; (4) mostly yes; (5) yes

_____ 1. Did I arrange to be uninterrupted?
_____ 2. Did I make us both as comfortable as possible?
_____ 3. Did I make and maintain eye contact?
_____ 4. Did I explore his/her feelings?
_____ 5. Did I substantiate my statements with specific incidents, facts?
_____ 6. Did I check to be sure he/she understood?
_____ 7. Did I listen to him/her?
_____ 8. Did I state the problem(s) clearly?
_____ 9. Did I challenge him/her to further growth?
_____ 9b. Did I help him/her formulate a growth plan?
_____ 10. Does he/she understand my expectations?
_____ 11. Did I maintain control of the session?
_____ 12. Was the session too long or too short?

*Copyrighted by Supportive Management/Educational Services (SMES), Milwaukee, Wisc., 1978.

The variation in performance appraisal forms is infinite. To be useful, the form should include four factors: (1) a picture of the employee including strengths and growth needs, (2) the past year's history of performance, (3) an appraisal of the individual's value to the organization, and (4) the plan for development for the coming year.

The performance appraisal session is designed for mutual discussion and exploration. The two involved persons meet as equals; each brings a set of data, expectations, impressions, and expertise. The session is one of joint planning, involving such decisions as: What shall be the goal? How shall it be approached? What role will each party play? To be avoided are threats, ultimatums, rationalizations, and secret stored-up observations.

For many supervisors, the one-to-one session is fraught with anxiety. This is also true for the subordinate. Additionally, the negative connotations and unhealthy practices often connected with performance appraisal make this a stressful meeting. The questionnaire above implies methods, arrangements, and behaviors that may minimize the negative effects and aftereffects of the process.

Delegation

Delegation is probably the most poorly used tool available to the supervisor. Delegation is a general form of directing based on (1) personal philosophy, (2) abilities of co-workers, and (3) organization policies. Tasks best delegated are those utilizing all persons' capabilities; they should be assigned to the person with most expertise or to one who is seeking growth opportunities. Too often tasks are delegated either because they are unpleasant or for expedience to persons who are available, liked least, willing, or passive. Appropriate delegation will result in personnel development in skill, confidence, knowledge, and recognition. Supervisors are sometimes hesitant to delegate because they lose control, recognition, and indispensability; these are frightening losses to many. However, delegation also presents supervisors with new opportunities, with free time to accomplish new projects or to catch up.

Delegating in a growth-producing manner begins with self-assessment and self-growth. To delegate effectively the supervisor must have in-depth knowledge of the people and the task. In order to improve the delegation pattern, the supervisor must be aware of past and present practices. To ensure the best possible results of delegation, the supervisor must be specific in giving instructions, concentrating on clear, concise, and complete communication. To facilitate staff development, the supervisor needs to keep informed, examine progress reports, and offer feedback and suggestions.

Decision making

Decision making involves a series of steps:
1. Definition, description of the situation
2. Generation of ideas
3. Evaluation of alternatives
4. Choice of alternative
5. Implementation of choice
6. Evaluation of choice

Vroom and Yetton* have established a method of deciding that is dependent on quality, commitment, and time. A decision can be made rapidly by oneself if one has sufficient information and can be fairly sure subordinates will comply. Decision making has been reduced to a mechanical science: define the situation, gather solutions, weigh the pros and cons of each, choose, go with it. And yet . . .

Involvement (or lack of it) in decision making is one of the most common job dissatisfiers, demoralizers, and frequent causes of job turnover. Adults like to feel they have some control over themselves and their job situations. People are more committed to decisions in which they have a part. Involving persons in each or any of the steps in decision making results in staff development, team development, commitment, job satisfaction, better quality decisions, and improved morale. It may take more time.

Problem solving

Problem solving has many of the attributes and characteristics of decision making. However, whereas decisions can be proactive and stem from desire for growth, problem solving tends to be reactive and to have its roots in dis-

*See Chapter 2, Ref. 18.

cord. Supervisors can deal with problems by withdrawing, smoothing, dominating, compromising, or confronting. Withdrawing is least effective and consists of ignoring the problem or the person. This practice results in barrier formation and loss of subordinate respect. Smoothing, minimizing the problem, and giving in to easy solutions will only cover the roots of the problem, causing it to reoccur. This frequently results in loss of face and feelings of frustration coming from subordinates. Dominating is the practice of solving problems through use of power (yours or a higher manager). This results in resistance, hurt feelings, and divisions. Compromising involves each part giving in a little with the result that everyone is somewhat dissatisfied and no one is fully committed to the solution. Confronting the problem consists of exploring both (all) viewpoints of the problem, redefining the problem, identifying roots of the problem, sharing ownership of the problem, and resolving it. It results in team and individual growth, and in creative solutions. It also requires the most supervisory skill.

Helping relationship skills

"The practice of *helping* is not a cloak to be put on or taken off; it is a way of being, a set of beliefs, an atmosphere or attitude projected. Helping involves a set of skills and behaviors that are integral to one's interactions."[20] Helping includes the following behaviors:

- Awareness—recognizing fragile behavior changes, sensing alterations in interactions
- Acceptance—genuine feelings of interest, liking, empathy, and caring
- Investment—reaching out, acknowledging one's awareness, acceptance, and availability
- Facilitation—unbiased attentiveness while others express their concerns
- Mobilization—probing for insights, new awareness, a change from circular thinking
- Assistance—help with the plan developed by the help seeker, roles that are helpful but do not take over
- Looking back—assessing past performance, honing one's skills as a helper

The form on p. 102 provides self-assessment of requisite helping skills. Examining oneself and then seeking feedback from another relative to these skills will provide the supervisor a picture of self as helper.

SUPERVISING TO RETAIN SELF

Much of the onus for retention of staff nurses and nurses in general has been correctly placed on the supervisor. We have examined many of the skills, roles, styles, beliefs, responsibilities, and challenges of the supervisor in this regard. It is also important for the supervisor to fulfill job duties in a

manner that allows him or her to continue in the role or the profession.
Supervisors are just as prone to burnout as are any other employee. The supervisor has four critical indexes that portend turnover (either in fact or in withdrawal).

Frustration

The nursing supervisor was originally trained to be a bedside caregiver.
Feelings of self-worth, job satisfaction, and sense of self came from patients,

HIGH-LEVEL HUMAN RELATING BEHAVIORS

Listed below are a number of behaviors that are essential to high-level human relating. Rate yourself on these behaviors, using the following scale.

1	2	3	4	5	6	7	8	9
Very weak		**Moderately weak**		**Adequate**		**Moderately strong**		**Very strong**

Note that a rating of 5 means that in a particular category you would consider yourself a *resource* person (if only minimally so) in a human relationship or a group, a *giver* in that category rather than just a receiver.

_____ **Empathy:** I see the world through the eyes of others. I understand others because I can get inside the skin of others. I listen well to all the cues (both verbal and nonverbal) that the other emits, and I respond to these cues.

_____ **Warmth, respect:** I express (and not just feel) in a variety of ways that I am "for" others, that I respect them. I accept others even though I do not necessarily approve of what they do. I am an *actively* supportive person.

_____ **Genuineness:** I am genuine rather than phony in my interactions. I do not hide behind roles or facades. Others know where I stand. I am myself in my interactions.

_____ **Concreteness:** I am not vague when I speak to others. I do not speak in generalities nor do I beat around the bush. I deal with concrete experience and behavior when I talk. I am direct and specific.

_____ **Initiative:** In my relationships I act rather than just react. I go out to contact others without waiting to be contacted. I am spontaneous. I take initiative over a wide variety of ways of relating to others. When in a group I "own" the interactions that take place between other members, and get involved in them.

_____ **Immediacy:** I deal openly and directly with my relationships to others. I know where I stand with others and they know where they stand with me because I deal with the relationship.

_____ **Self-disclosure:** I let others know the "person inside." I am not exhibitionistic, but I use self-disclosure to help establish sound relationships with others. I am open without being a "secret revealer" or a "secret-searcher," for I am important, not just my secrets.

_____ **Feelings and emotions:** I am not afraid to deal directly with emotion, my own or others'; in my relationships I allow myself both to feel and to give expression to what I feel. I expect others to do the same, but I do not "inflict" my emotions on others.

_____ **Confrontation:** I challenge others' responsibility and with care. I use confrontation as a way of getting involved with others; I do not use confrontation to punish.

_____ **Self-exploration:** I examine my life-style and behavior and want others to help me to do so. I respond to confrontation as nondefensively as possible; I am open to changing my behavior. I use confrontation as an opportunity for self-exploration.

Modified from Egan, G.: Face to face, Monterey, Calif., 1973, Brooks-Cole Publishing Co.

patients' families, and hands-on exercise. The supervisor works through others; the jobs from the past are experienced vicariously or not at all. There are, of course, other rewards in supervision. The transition from one reward system to another is a difficult one, not supported by the profession (or your neighbors), and is impossible for some nurses. Good bedside nurses are often promoted to supervisory positions; it is found that "external rewards draw a person to a job, but internal rewards keep him [her] there and stimulate him [her] to do good work."[11]

A useful exercise for the supervisor is to brainstorm the tasks that are personally rewarding. Rank the top 10. On a second sheet rank these same 10 by organization reward. Compare the two lists to ascertain your frustration index.

	My reward	Organization reward	Frustration index
Staffing	5	1	4
Attending meetings	4	2	2
Counseling employees	2	4	2
Teaching	3	3	0
Patient care	1	5	4

Frustration indexes of 4 or over identify areas that require attention. The supervisor can change her orientation, work out a different arrangement with the organization, be frustrated, be reassigned, or resign (turnover).

Isolation

Nursing supervisors have fewer peers than do staff nurses. They often feel isolated, lonely, misunderstood, and without help. The transition from staff to supervisor is complete when one is able to view other supervisors (previous superordinates) as confidants, peers, and resources. A peer support group is extremely worthwhile for the supervisor. Unlike the floor nurses, the supervisor's domain is removed from that of peers. Consequently, interactions and communication with peers require effort.

Self-worth

Much of the supervisor's work is not visible; it takes place in planning, gathering data, making decisions, and presenting information. Few subordinates are aware of these efforts, and fewer still actively or openly value them. Supervisors expend much energy on problem solving for a subordinate or a unit, altering schedules to meet others' needs, and working for others. It is possible to lose track of one's identity.

Supervisors must take some time for themselves. They need to plan for *their* career, *their* vacation, *their* professional growth and stimulation, and *their* self-assessment. Supervisors are motivated too by self-esteem and self-actualization. It is imperative that there be time for these needs to be identified and met.

Facilitation toll

A facilitator is one who assists the progress of another, an intervening agent through which an effect is produced. The supervisor is a facilitator, one who makes arrangements so another can provide direct health care. The supervisor runs interference to allow for optimum circumstances, and makes sacrifices (that cost time, effort, and often worry) to make work pleasant. The role of helper, giver, vehicle, or facilitator—often unseen and unappreciated—is very draining. This person needs a resource, a source, as Norma Lang says, "to fill up his/her bucket."

A CONCEPTUAL CONCLUSION

"Performing well as a first level supervisor is like walking the circus high wire. In both positions, the ability to maintain one's balance when shifting forces pull in opposite directions is a measure of one's success."[16] Supervisors have varied responsibilities, utilize a variety of styles, are responsible for building a team, regulate socialization issues, must develop certain skills and abilities, and need to be self-preserving. But how does a successful supervisor behave?

Sasser and Leonard [16] consolidated much research to describe effective supervisors. They take pride in their work, are quite critical, do not always like their job, solicit subordinates' opinions, evaluate subordinates frequently, and encourage and praise subordinates. Successful supervisors are believed to have influence in the organization; they are able to supply subordinates with information, supplies, and equipment; they spend time in meetings with employees and give general rather than specific instructions. Good supervisors view employees as individuals, are quick to reward, are more apt to check the activity than the location of employees. "A successful supervisor seems to have the ability to balance the demands of task, employees, union, and management with his/her own needs for esteem and respect. But this balancing act takes place in a ring where not all of these demands can be met at once."[16] At this time in the history of health care, the supervisor supervising for retention must reassess the demands of task, organization, union, and management against the demands of the practicing nurse because the past "balancing" has caused turnover, burnout, and exit from the profession.

REFERENCES AND ADDITIONAL READINGS

1. Argyris, C.: The incompleteness of social psychological theory: examples from small group, cognitive consistency, and attribution research, New Haven, Conn., 1970, Department of Administrative Sciences, Yale University.
2. Blake, R.R., and Mouton, J.S.: The new managerial grid, Houston, 1978, Gulf Publishing Co.
3. Colby, J.D., and Wallace, R.L.: Performance appraisal: help or hindrance to employee productivity? Personnel Administrator **20:**37-39, Oct. 1975.

4. Dyer, W.G.: Team building: issues and alternatives, Reading, Mass., 1978, Addison-Wesley Publishing Co.
5. Egan, G.: Face to face, Monterey, Calif., 1973, Brooks-Cole Publishing Co.
6. Franklin, W.H., Jr.: What Japanese managers know that American managers don't, Admin. Mgmt. **42**(9):38, Sept. 1981.
7. Hall, J., and Donnell, S.M.: Managerial achievement: the personal side of behavioral theory, Human Relations **32**(1):77-101, 1979.
8. Hampton, D.R.: Contemporary management, New York, 1981, McGraw-Hill Book Co.
9. Harvey, J.: The Abilene paradox: the management of agreement, Organizational Dynamics **3**(1):63-80, Summer 1974.
10. Likert, R.: New patterns in management, New York, 1961, McGraw-Hill Book Co.
11. McCloskey, J.: Influence of rewards and incentives on staff nurse turnover rate, Nurs. Res. **23**(3):246, May-June 1974.
12. McGregor, D.: The human side of enterprise, New York, 1960, McGraw-Hill Book Co.
13. Miles, R.E.: Theories of management, New York, 1975, McGraw-Hill Book Co.
14. Ouchi, W.: Theory Z, New York, 1981, Avon Books.
15. Reilly, A.J., and Jones, J.E.: Team building, Ann. Hdbk. Group Facilitators **4**:228; 230, 1974.
16. Sasser, W.E., and Leonard, F.S.: Let first level supervisors do their job, Harvard Bus. Rev. **58**(2):113;117, March-April 1980.
17. Schein, E.: Organizational socialization, the third Douglas Murray McGregor Memorial Lecture of the Alfred P. Sloan School of Management, Massachusetts Institute of Technology, Cambridge, Oct. 1967.
18. Tannenbaum, R., and Schmidt, W.H.: How to choose a leadership pattern, Harvard Bus. Rev. **51**(3):167, May-June 1973.
19. Thurkettle, M.A., and Jones, S.L.: Conflict as a systems process: theory and management, J. Nurs. Admin. **8**(1):40, Jan. 1978.
20. Vogt, J.F., and Velthouse, B.A.: Collegial helping, unpublished article, 1982.

4

MOTIVATION

FRAMEWORK CONSIDERATIONS
Motivation is individual

Motivation is inherently individual. This simple concept when applied to the problem of nurse turnover will make a difference. Over the past 40 years there has been a burgeoning of motivation theories and research findings—significant contributions to helping us understand the very complex issue of motivation. But in the last analysis, we must return to the basics; that is, motivational considerations must be applied and reapplied, formed and re-formed to provide the key to motivating each person. Recent theoretical constructs and research information have provided more data—more excellent grist—for tapping individual potential in behalf of the organization.

The responsibility for motivation

Motivation is an organizational and personal responsibility (see Fig. 4-1). It is most effective when the process of designing motivation strategies includes representatives of each group. Where the shared honing of such strategies is viewed as an *ongoing healthy process*, it will contribute to the motivational concerns as much as the outcomes themselves do. It must be perceived, and in actuality *be*, that people are working together to meet the congruent needs requisite for personal contribution to organizational effectiveness.

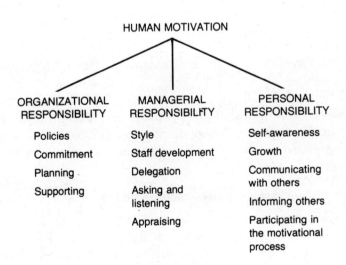

HUMAN MOTIVATION

ORGANIZATIONAL RESPONSIBILITY	MANAGERIAL RESPONSIBILITY	PERSONAL RESPONSIBILITY
Policies	Style	Self-awareness
Commitment	Staff development	Growth
Planning	Delegation	Communicating with others
Supporting	Asking and listening	Informing others
	Appraising	Participating in the motivational process

FIG. 4-1
Human motivation.

Personal and organizational life

Why is motivation so important? Perhaps the reason is that the primary elements related to motivation are so pervasive to human existence in today's world:

1. The human condition is to *strive* constantly—most often toward growth, toward a productive, useful, meaningful life—for greater self-worth.

2. Therefore more people work outside of the domestic setting today than ever before, including men, women, single, married, old, young, black, white, red, yellow. We have many more variables to contend with and to develop from than in our past history.

3. Organizations have *behavioral requirements* for people: employees must join the organization; employees must remain with the organization; and employees must transcend "dependable" role performance to creative, spontaneous, and innovative behavior at work.

4. The very survival of organizations is directly influenced by and directly influences motivational factors. The relationship between organizational functioning and the behavior of people is more obvious and necessary to understand than ever before.

5. There are more and more constraints placed on organizational operations: unions, government regulations, increased competition. As a result, the emphasis must now turn from "more" to "better"—to the maximum utilization of all resources, including our human resources.

6. Human resources can be developed within the organizational framework. Those who stay contribute to organizational stability and productivity; those who learn and grow contribute to the enhancement of organizational effectiveness.

7. And the growth takes us back to our starting point: the human condition is to strive, to grow toward *contributing* for an increased sense of self-worth.

Fig. 4-2 helps define the cyclical nature of these factors as they relate to current human conditions. It demonstrates and identifies the synergistic relationship necessary to the development of personal and organizational systems. Synergy is the motivational hope for nursing, nurses, hospitals, and health care.

The relationships among motivation, productivity, and retention

Motivation is directly related to productivity and retention. It is this research-supported perspective from which the retention of nurses must be examined. In today's work world, where concerns regarding productivity abound and in hospitals where nursing turnover runs rampant, this theoretical linkage can make a significant, positive impact. (As it is now, this linkage is

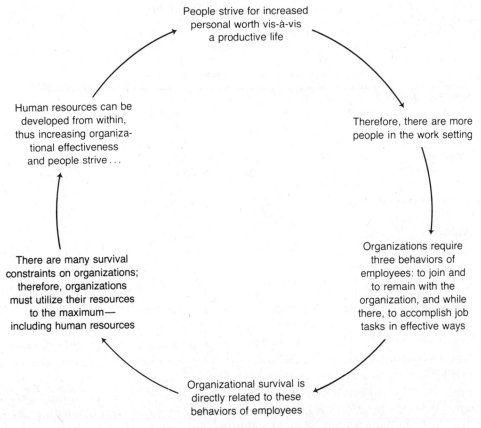

FIG. 4-2
A cyclical model of motivational forces operating in today's world.

most often working against nurses, nursing, and hospitals.) Although we are most interested here in the retention of nurses, let us not forget the other half of the relationship, that is, productivity. Contemporary motivational models have had as a major goal the diagnosis and alleviation of two concomitant problems: low retention and low productivity.

Retention from the staff nurse's viewpoint: motivational forces

In the final analysis, retention is an individual matter. This is not to deny the contribution of research that has summarized data relevant to retention and that has allowed generalities regarding retention to be devised and examined. But, as in the case of motivation, we must understand the very personal nature of retention. There are motivational forces that affect each person's decision to remain with or to leave an organization. It is important to remember, however, that because a certain force may promote retention, its polar

TABLE 4-1
Force-field analysis of possible forces examined by nurses
deciding to remain in or leave their present places of employment

	Driving forces		Restraining forces	
Within nurse	Strong personal work values and goals Requisite abilities and traits		Weak performance-reward linkage Lack of job involvement	
Within all management levels	Perceptions of equitable treatment	Quasi-equilibrium	Distrust of management	**GOAL: DECISION TO STAY OR LEAVE**
Within the job	Role clarity		Desire to have control over one's job	
Within the organization	Valued rewards contingent on performance		Potential rewards appealing	

opposite would not necessarily prompt leaving an organization. We must not fall into the trap of making simplistic assumptions such as this. One way to demonstrate this concept is to borrow the idea of Richard Steers in his book on organizational behavior.[19] Steers has utilized Kurt Lewin's force-field analysis technique to examine a variety of forces affecting productivity. Table 4-1 presents selected driving and restraining motivational forces each staff nurse who works in hospital (organizational) settings might weigh in making the decision to remain with or leave the facility. This means of presenting motivational factors illustrates that a nurse actually weighs positive *and* negative forces in making decisions. It also indicates to those responsible for examining "the facts" the importance of the two sets of data to problem resolution. (A more in-depth description of the force-field analysis and its relationship to the change process is presented on pp. 240-241 of Chapter 8.) The specific motivational factors identified in Table 4-1 have been generally agreed on as those having a significant impact on nurses' decisions to stay.

The staff nurse is complex. His or her decision to stay or leave is more likely a constellation of many forces. We must, in our analysis of motivation's role in retention, remember the individual. We must examine all forces and not shortchange a human being in terms of the motivational pressures affecting work life choices.

THREE OVERLOOKED THEORIES OF MOTIVATION
Expectancy-valence theory, expanded

In the 1930s and 1940s, Kurt Lewin and Edward Tolman were strongly involved in research and activities that recognize two major components of human behavior:

1. Individual characteristics (personality traits, attitudes, needs, values)
2. The perceived environment

According to their work, human behavior results from the *interaction* of these two variables. Thus

Human behavior = f (Individual characteristics + Perceived environment)

The framework for this perspective was Kurt Lewin's field theory. Lewin theorized that one's behavior was based on one's "life space." This life space was composed of the individual's perceptual field plus one's environmental field. Lewin, in devising his model, included a variety of mathematical constructs and symbols to illustrate the "dynamic" qualities of his theory—his primary point being that there was a differentiation between the individual and his or her environment, and that the different parts were in constantly changing constellations. Lewin showed the force, elements, and weight of each element affected in a pictorial representation, often utilizing *vectors* to demonstrate directionality. Lewin's theory also included the point that these factors were never unmoving; what may be heavily weighted at one time, may not be at another. Each of the boundary lines identified in the life-space model (see Fig. 4-3) is fluid. It is the individual's ultimate goal, however, to reach equilibrium; thus one constantly brings energy, tension, value ("force") to one's behavior. It is this force that motivates (and that prompts) behavior change; one increases one's emotions, activities, needs, information, social relationships, thus changing the makeup of the life space. A person is motivated by growth and by development, through enhancement.

Dr. Allen Menlo,[12] a professor at the University of Michigan, has for many years influenced his students by introducing a somewhat more complex equation for understanding human behavior, motivation, and behavior change.

$$\text{Behavior change} = f\left(\frac{\text{One's perception of self + One's perceptions of friendly forces}}{\text{One's perceptions of unfriendly forces}}\right)$$

According to this framework, there are two key components: a person's self-concept and perceptions of the forces around one's self. (Though a perceptual model at its core, this view integrates Carl Roger's postulates concerning the individual's self-regard as a motivator.)

The key component of the above discussion is one's *perceptions*. The key principle is that for a person to be motivated, changes in that person's perceptions must occur. Focuses of change efforts to effect motivation include:

- Values, attitudes, traits, needs
- Self-perceptions
- The environment

We believe that activities in each of these areas are motivational and can increase nurse retention. It is upon this "perceptual foundation" that expec-

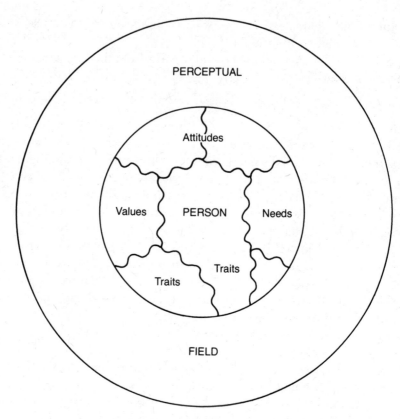

FIG. 4-3
A pictorial representation of Kurt Lewin's concept: life space.

tancy-valence theories of motivation are based. In short, one's perceptions determine one's expectations. Clifton Williams[24] has defined the two prime terms as follows:

- *Expectancy* refers to a person's judgment of the likelihood that a specific outcome will follow a specific course of action.
- *Valence* refers to the value a person places on a particular outcome (consequence of an action).

Likelihood of the outcome plus the outcome's value—it is the combined effect of these two variables that affects motivation. High expectancy without high valency will not motivate, and vice versa. Both are necessary in order to motivate.

Motivational force = Expectancy × Valence

In the 1960s, Victor Vroom[23] expanded and popularized expectancy theory. He identified three factors:

1. Effort-performance (E-P): The relationship between the amount of effort expended and performance (defined as attainment of objectives)
2. Performance-outcome (P-O): the relationship between the level of performance and the outcome (usually a reward)
3. Valence of outcome (V): the value of the outcome

As expressed earlier, each of these components is critical to motivation; therefore expectancy theory is a relationship theory and must be expressed as follows:

E-P		P-O		V		M
Expectancy that performance is possible	×	Expectancy that reward will result	×	Value of reward	=	Motivation

Summary and implications. This discussion has identified four integral sources crucial to the process of motivation:

1. The person
2. The person's self-concept
3. The person's expectations
4. The environment

A change in one of the variables will lead to a change in the others as well as in the individual's motivation. It is imperative that motivation efforts implemented to enhance the retention factor not ignore this concept of interrelatedness. These activities must enhance each of the four areas simultaneously with careful attention being paid to the sequencing and results of each activity undertaken.

For example, let us assume that one of our strategies to promote motivation (and to affect retention positively) is to provide a series of "personal growth classes" for staff nurses (i.e., *the person*). Let us also assume that this strategy is implemented before the organization (*the environment*) has examined its benefits package and designed improvements, or before head nurses have had first-line supervisory training—both of which are planned, but for later. But the person has changed (has new attitudes, values, needs) while the environment (supervisors, benefits) has not, during the same time period. The result may well be that the person will leave to accommodate his or her new "self" *before* the environment has been addressed. The choice, sequence, and timing are dependent on each separate organization: its persons, its circumstances, its history, its goals, its characteristics. Although inappropriate above, the same example may be the appropriate intervention means in another organization. A whole plan and careful assessment are imperative to increasing motivation vis-à-vis the expectation-valence (expanded) model; moreover, assessing and planning must be *ongoing* because people continue to grow, to develop, to change.

Specific activities are referred to and examined in depth throughout this

TABLE 4-2

Enhancement activities based on four motivational variables

Elements in the motivational process	Possible enhancement activities
THE PERSON	Values clarification activities, personal growth training, human relations training, feedback sessions
THE PERSON'S SELF-CONCEPT	Feedback → value activities, praise, self-appraisal activities, encouragement, promotion, special privileges
THE PERSON'S EXPECTATIONS	Data gathering and assessment by self and others of past experiences and expectations; behavioral change: personal or organizational; information-sharing sessions
THE ENVIRONMENT	Survey-research activities, management development, team building, new policies and procedures, organization design, first-line supervisory training, new benefits packages

book in relation to each component of motivation identified above. A brainstormed list that is somewhat representative is presented in Table 4-2. The possibilities are infinite; the process is unending and the outcomes are forever a challenge.

The Porter-Lawler theory of motivation

In 1968, Porter and Lawler[15] introduced a dynamic model that has come to be called the Porter-Lawler model of motivation. In actuality their model stems from and is often included within expectancy theories. What makes this model special is that it is functional in its specificity. The model identifies nine separate components relevant to the motivational *process,* each of which can be examined and changed (enhanced) to promote the desired outcomes. It also pictures motivation as an *ongoing* process allowing for growth, both personal and organizational. A diagram of their model is shown in Fig. 4-4. The numbers in the upper right-hand corners indicate the order or sequence of the process. According to Porter and Lawler, an individual's performance (6) is based on three ingredients:

1. Abilities and traits (4)
2. Role clarity and acceptance (5)
3. Opportunity to perform or to put forth effort (3)

These three ingredients (see Table 4-3) directly affect one's performance, although one's effort (3) is dependent on the likelihood that effort will lead to the rewards (2) and that those rewards are valued by the person (1). Accomplishment (6) results in rewards, be they intrinsic (7a) or extrinsic (7b) in nature. The dotted line between accomplishment (6) and perceived equitability

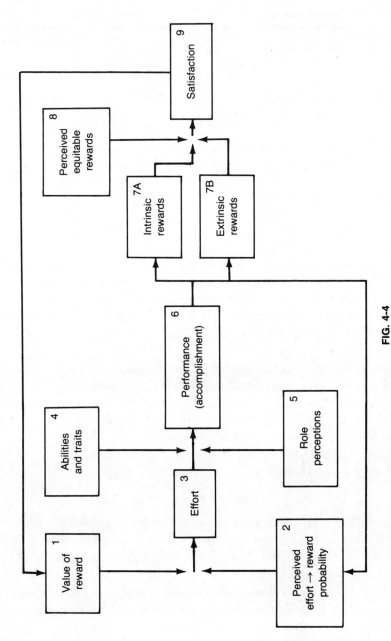

FIG. 4-4

The expectancy model of motivation. (From Porter, L.W., and Lawler, E.E. III: Managerial attitudes and performance, Homewood, Ill., © 1968, Dorsey-Irwin, Inc.)

TABLE 4-3

Key elements in three of the variables affecting human performance

Variables affecting performance	Key elements in each
ABILITIES AND TRAITS	Intellectual capabilities (verbal comprehension, inductive reasoning, memory) Technical skills and knowledge (job related) Personal traits (complexity)
ROLE CLARITY AND ACCEPTANCE	Increases amount of energy directed toward work goals Increases commitment to work goals Increases involvement in one's job Increases job satisfaction Increases work group cohesiveness
EFFORT	Opportunity to perform must not be unduly restrained Control of production can lead to quality changes but not quantity of output changes

of the rewards (8) means that each individual is the sole judge of whether the rewards received are equitable. (It is this concept on which the equity theory, which follows in this section, is based.) Satisfaction (9) results from rewards (7) and their perceived equity. It is this satisfaction that helps the person determine how valuable the reward is (1), which in turn affects future performance.

A major implication of this model is that *job performance leads to satisfaction*. A sense of achievement is the basis for motivation; one who is motivated in terms of this model is satisfied and is therefore more likely to be retained within the organization. Successful job performance is based on both the individual and the environment as stated in Lewin's field theory. The implication is that both individual and environmental components can be integrated into a system that is mutually beneficial.

Equity theory

Adams[1] in the early 1960s recognized the importance of other human beings in the process of motivation. Though his theory is far more simplistic than the two theories discussed heretofore, it appears to have profound implications for the professional nurse. The basic premise is that the individual objectively or subjectively determines a ratio of his or her job inputs to job outcomes (Table 4-4), and then compares that ratio with reference persons. If there is an imbalance (inequity), the individual will experience psychological tension. The individual will constantly work to reduce such tension by achieving equity (or psychological balance). People can reduce the inequity by one of two means: (1) changing their effort level or (2) changing the nature

TABLE 4-4

Job inputs and outcomes

Job inputs	Job outcomes
Effort	Pay
Skills	Promotion
Education	Recognition
Performance	Achievement
	Status

of the reward. The concept of equity can result in increasing or reducing one's efforts to bring them into line with referent persons or groups.

In 1965 Adams identified six methods individuals utilize to reduce inequity:

1. Alter the quality or quantity of their input.
2. Alter the outcomes.
3. Cognitively distort inputs or outcomes.
4. Leave the job.
5. Distort the inputs or outcomes of others.
6. Change the sources of reference.

Individuals are hardworking; the amount of energy they have, however, is limited. The more fair the circumstances of work, the more likely their energy bank can be utilized in behalf of their work; the more unfair these circumstances, the greater the personal tension, thus the more energy must be put into reducing the psychological tension they experience.

A study conducted in 1970 by Telly et al.[22] found that turnover was directly related to equity. In the job setting experiencing high turnover, hourly employees had higher perceptions of inequity than those who worked in a job setting experiencing low tension. In this study, variables subject to the "equity test" included:

- Supervision
- Working conditions
- Intrinsic rewards
- Social aspects of the job

It is important to point out that most of the research on equity theory over the past 15 years has concentrated on pay levels (outcomes). Pay, being a basic need of hourly workers, has been the logical starting point. Without exception, the basic tenets of equity theory have been supported in relationship to pay levels. It is important to note that research indicates that the equity theory of motivation is especially valid for women in the work force. It is this combination of pay plus women vis-à-vis equity that has a high degree of relevance for the retention of professional nurses.

Finally, in research conducted in 1978, evidence was gleaned showing that women at work perceived inequities related to the following variables listed from the highest perceived inequity variable to the lowest)[16]:

- Pay
- Job/skills fit
- Access to informal communication or sources of information relevant to job
- Expectations to do more work, different work, or less prestigious work
- Affirmative action guidelines
- Access to in-house training programs
- Informal social activities

This particular research provides rich data for the hospital organization seeking to retain its professional nurses. Though direct implications can be drawn, the most important recognitions are that the equity-inequity theory is relevant, especially for women in the work force; further, the variables identified by each person are *individual* in nature and therefore must be individually identified for the purpose of resolution—for the purpose of retention.

Implications: for the individual, the manager(s), the organization

The first part of this chapter examined the responsibility for motivation, indicating that success requires a three-pronged effort: organizational, managerial, personal. The theoretical constructs explored to this point clearly support this tenet. Table 4-5 shows the relationship and indicates several implications for each component in the motivational scheme of things. The listing on the far right is meant to identify behaviors but is not meant to be exhaustive. Many nurses, nurse-managers, and administrators in organizations have been making strides in the "right direction" without having the benefits of theoretical support. Motivation theory has grown far beyond the early "fear" and "needs" orientations. Our hope is that by highlighting expectancy-valence theory (including field theory and self-concept precepts), the Porter-Lawler model, and equity theory, we have added more relevant, applicable concepts that will lend themselves to the development of creative, effective, and lasting nurse retention plans, strategies, and activities. We suggest that as organizations and persons undertake the positive step of increasing nurse retention, they utilize the design model espoused in Table 4-5 especially for their early brainstorming phases. In representative group settings, (1) write down the various and significant elements of a theory, (2) consider the organizational implications for *your* organization, (3) and (4) identify managerial and then personal implications for your institution. Repeat steps (2) through (4) for each theory. The resultant data will provide a firm ground for increasing the retention of professional nurses. Incidentally, management has been identified throughout as a single group: this is an over-

TABLE 4-5
Organizational, managerial, and personal implications of motivation theories

Theoretical orientation	Focus of responsibility	Types and examples of responsibilities
EXPECTANCY-VALENCE THEORY, EXPANDED	Organizational	Conduct ongoing climate assessment surveys; clearly define work roles and job task systems; base reward system on performance; issue a mission statement recognizing employee contributions.
	Managerial	Give coaching and guidance; provide immediate and specific feedback on job activities, matching employee desires with organizational rewards; recognize the subjectivity and individuality of personal reward preferences; demonstrate that effort will lead to preferred reward; recognize role in how employees see themselves.
	Personal	Enhance one's capabilities through skill development; examine one's self in terms of attitudes and needs; value one's self; know one's value system and its relation to work; recognize that one's self-worth is affected by the effort-reward relationship.
PORTER-LAWLER MODEL	Organizational	Provide various technical and personal growth opportunities; interface system, job descriptions, and relationships; base recruitment, selection, and placement procedures on "fit"; encourage innovative sharing and self-control in manager-employee relationships; include employees and actively advocate their role defining the nature of the work environment.
	Managerial	Recognize that satisfied workers are those who expend great effort in task accomplishment; provide each employee with tasks that encourage stretching behaviors; be willing to clarify role and job expectations; provide employees with control over their own performance environment; include employees in assessing and structuring the work environment.
	Personal	Seek ongoing personal and professional development; examine one's value system vis-à-vis rewards and make them known; understand and accept requirements of the job.

Continued.

TABLE 4-5—cont'd

Organizational, managerial, and personal implications of motivation theories

Theoretical orientation	Focus of responsibility	Types and examples of responsibilities
EQUITY THEORY	Organizational	Clearly define salary structure; base system of distribution of rewards on equity; maintain a fair and consistent performance appraisal system and forms; be aware of market standards; have a monitoring device for recognizing significant changes in the input/outcomes ratio; recognize that distribution of rewards is seen as a social responsibility.
	Managerial	Demonstrate willingness to explain differences in inequities; recognize the importance of perception in employee motivation; constantly assess your perceptions of the work place in relation to workers' perceptions; be willing to correct any real inequities; confront inaccurate perceptions of inequities.
	Personal	Be honest with self; examine carefully feelings of inequity; recognize the impact of feelings of inequity on one's job performance; recognize the importance of one's perceptions on motivations; do not devalue one's feelings of unfairness; be open to information demonstrating inequity and equity.

simplification. Management may include hospital administrators, nursing administrators, middle management (such as supervisors, assistant directors), and first-line supervisors (head nurses). It is imperative that *each* group/level look at itself in light of its responsibilities in the motivation of nurses.

TWO PLUS THEORIES OF MOTIVATION THAT STARTED IT ALL
Theory X and theory Y

In 1960 in the book, *The Human Side of Enterprise*, Douglas McGregor[10] introduced his now famous conceptualization of managerial beliefs about employees: theory X and theory Y. His concepts did not represent the basis for a motivational theory per se. They did, however, have profound implications for managerial style and organizational climate, policies, and responsibilities as they affect employee motivation. Though often the focus is on the manager's relationship with employees, it is necessary also to give equal attention to the organization's relationship with the employee.

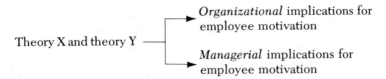

Theory X and theory Y —
- *Organizational* implications for employee motivation
- *Managerial* implications for employee motivation

Over the years, most practitioners have examined theory X and Y postures primarily focusing on their relevancy for managers (and usually their shortcomings at that.) It is imperative that the focus here be on the *environment* in which both managers *and* employees operate. The self-fulfilling prophecy concept must be recognized as it relates to the organization's impact on employee behaviors and managerial activities. The organization should be treated as an entity *separate* from its leadership as Douglas McGregor's unique and most significant contributions to motivation are examined.

McGregor, in his attempts to improve productivity in organizations, recognized that people, in their attempts to influence human activity within the work setting, appeared to operate from two distinct and opposite postures.* Upon closer observation and thought, he perceived that the influencers had two different sets of assumptions about people. He called these sets of assumptions theory X and theory Y, and he applied these labels to managers (e.g., a theory X manager). These labels can also be applied to organizations (e.g., a theory Y organization). Both managerial style *and* organizational environment can be examined and understood in light of these underlying assumptions about people. Managerial (and organizational) effectiveness conceivably rests within the usually unconscious effects of these basic assumptions on people's actions. It is these actions that in turn are most often translated into motivational methodologies. According to Mescon et al.,[14] the underlying assumptions directly determine the need (lower level or higher order needs) to which the manager and/or organization appeals.

Specifically, McGregor called the "traditional" assumptions about people theory X; he referred to those assumptions steeped in the more recent behavioral and social science knowledge as theory Y. These assumptions are listed in Table 4-6 in McGregor's words.

In Robinson's compilation of Edgar Schein's perspectives, the theory X manager limits his or her motivational style, is inflexible, and has a predisposition toward utilizing autocratic and/or paternalistic decision-making methods. Such managers focus on lower level human needs and tend to see an employee as a replaceable cog in the productivity conveyor belt. These managers highly structure their employees' work. In addition, they seldom involve their employees in any phase of the decision-making process. The

*Throughout this discussion, McGregor's X and Y distinctions are referred to as discrete concepts. However, it is important to remember that in reality persons tend to operate from some *combination* of theory X and theory Y constructs.

most common motivational style is the utilization of psychological pressure (usually in the form of threats). Theory X managers most often act as though their views toward people are accurate and require no further examination. The above discussion focuses on the "hard" approach to managing, but the theory X manager may also utilize the "soft" approach. From this perspective, the manager still perceives employees as lazy, while believing the way to get

TABLE 4-6
Theory X and theory Y assumptions

Theory X	Theory Y
1. The average human being has an inherent dislike of work and will avoid it if possible.	1. The expenditure of physical and mental effort in work is as natural as play or rest. The average human being does not inherently dislike work. Depending on controllable conditions, work may be a source of satisfaction (and will be voluntarily performed) or a source of punishment (and will be avoided if possible).
2. Because of this characteristic dislike of work, most people must be coerced, controlled, directed, threatened with punishment to get them to put forth adequate effort toward the achievement of organizational objectives.	2. External control and the threat of punishment are not the only means of bringing about effort toward organizational objectives. People will exercise self-direction and self-control in the service of objectives to which they are committed.
3. The average human being prefers to be directed, wishes to avoid responsibility, has relatively little ambition, wants security above all.	3. Commitment to objectives is a function of the rewards associated with their achievement. The most significant of such rewards, e.g., the satisfaction of ego and self-actualization needs, can be direct products of effort directed toward organizational objectives.
	4. The average human being learns, under proper conditions, not only to accept but to seek responsibility. Avoidance of responsibility, lack of ambition, and emphasis on security are generally consequences of experiences, not inherent human characteristics.
	5. The capacity to exercise a relatively high degree of imagination, ingenuity, and creativity in the solution of organizational problems is widely, not narrowly, distributed in the population.
	6. Under the conditions of modern industrial life, the intellectual potentialities of the average human being are only partially utilized.

Source: McGregor, D.: The human side of enterprise, New York, 1960, McGraw-Hill Book Co.

them to work is to "be nice to them," to coax productive activity from them.[17] It is this attitudinal posture that is so demeaning in terms of human worth. Another less obvious theory X style is that of "benevolent autocracy." The autocrat in this case avoids the negative, coercive activities in favor of rewarding for "correct or good" behavior. Though authoritarian, this manager shows concern for the feelings and well-being of employees. However, the benevolent autocrat retains power through autonomous decision making and through the rigid structuring of work, as well as the enforcing of rules that limit employee behavior.

Theory X organizations have distinct characteristics. Such organizations tend to have few motivational alternatives. They tend to be run from the "top-down," emphasizing highly paternalistic and centralized decision making. Organizational strategies for motivating tend to be limited to monies and benefits, replacing employees if these are not enough. Top management groups or individuals seldom explore their own roles, behaviors, and policies when examining "motivational problems" within the organization. It is theory X hospital organizations that most often experience high turnover.

The theory Y manager, as his or her basis of operation, *involves* others as much as the task, environmental circumstances, and situation allow. This style assumes and actively sets high standards for all employees; the manager's operational expectation is that the highest outcomes will be achieved. The theory Y manager is a risk taker who allows employees to develop, to grow, to experiment with new behaviors and attitudes in terms of success and productivity. This manager provides opportunities for, seeks, and values employee input. It is the sum total of this input that defines work norms, behaviors, roles, responsibilities, atmosphere, strengths, and limitations. This manager focuses on facilitating a process rather than directing people and activities. Employees work within a structure that permits them to develop and to accomplish work behaviors while feeling a sense of personal worth. Motivational forces are *within* this work-person relationship. Trying and testing are encouraged; errors are accepted as indicators of learning better ways to fulfill the job requirements. The theory Y organization tends to be in the forefront of efficiency and effectiveness; it tends to be constantly focusing on "what works best" (not "better"). The theory Y organization is innovative but "solid," characterized by high degrees of interrelatedness. There are high levels of risk taking occurring at all pressure points: technology, finances, interpersonal, and human. Theory Y hospital organizations tend to have high levels of retention among their professional nursing staffs.

Douglas McGregor's theoretical perspective has in its rather short history had a major impact on the world of work. It has given labels to help identify the negative, positive, pervasive, and insidious forces that affect work places. More importantly, the theory Y orientation of valuing participation and showing concern for worker morale has led to innumerable advances affecting motivation in the following areas[10]:

1. Delegation of authority and decision making
2. Expansion and enrichment of jobs
3. Increase in the variety of worker activities and responsibilities
4. Improvement of open and flowing organizational communication

Hospitals and health care managers will do well to examine their programs, relationships, attitudinal environment, and specific job activities considering (but not limited to) theory X and theory Y assumptions. As well, they must consider *forging* new strategies while accepting those advances generated to date by other types of industry (e.g., manufacturing, banking). Hospital managers and administrators who move forward in these ways can expect to win the cooperation and enthusiastic support of employees in achieving organizational goals.[4] Individual motivation and employee retention can be by-products that can have concrete, demonstrable payoffs for the organization.

Need hierarchy theory

In the 1940s, a clinical psychologist named Abraham Maslow translated his experiences into one of the most quoted and referred to theories of motivation ever conceived: the need hierarchy theory. Two major premises served as the starting point for understanding his social-behavioral perception of motivation:

1. Each human being has many needs and these needs serve as the cornerstones for experiencing life.
2. The human being is a dynamic "becoming" entity.

Maslow believed that human needs were inborn (and thus essential to existence). He hypothesized further, that these needs were hierarchical, based on normal development patterns—encouraged by outside forces and by the person's own capabilities, wits, and efforts. These needs are as follows:

- Physiological (e.g., food, water, air, rest)
- Safety (e.g., a safe and secure physical space and emotional environment; freedom from threat)
- Belongingness and love (e.g., interaction, acceptance, friendships, love)
- Esteem (e.g., worthy self-concept; recognition, attention, appreciation for contributions)
- Self-actualization (e.g., becoming; a combination of cognitive and aesthetic needs that assure self-fulfillment)

These needs, according to Maslow, tend to define the human being's growth from infancy to adulthood; however, at any one time in life, depending on internal and external conditions, one need may dominate and strongly influence behavior. Duality forms the basis for motivation: the *self*, which seeks new and/or peak experiences that are memorable and desirable thus developing or growing; and a healthy *culture* that fosters this universal need for self-actualization.

In his initial writings, Maslow focused on the self-actualizing need; he especially concentrated on characteristics of persons he described as self-actualizing (see outline on p. 126). In his later writings, however, Maslow emphasized that self-actualization was a *process of becoming*—of reaching, seeking, experiencing. He indicated that unlike the other four needs, when the self-actualizing need is fulfilled it prompts an *increase* in the potency of this need to motivate. Five general statements conclude this brief summary of Abraham Maslow's theoretical posture:

1. It is normal for persons to be partially satisfied and unsatisfied in all of the basic need areas at the same time.
2. Once satisfied, physiological, safety, and belongingness-love needs are no longer motivators; they do, however, tend to require fulfillment before the other two needs can act as motivators.
3. If belongingness-love needs are significantly thwarted at any time, a person may become maladjusted and develop pathological patterns.
4. Esteem and self-actualizing needs never stop motivating; desire for achievement and adequacy is continuous.
5. The average person is both conscious and unconscious of his or her needs.

What is the relationship of Maslow's work to business, management, organizations? First, it is necessary to translate Maslow's concepts into work world applications. Judy Vogt, in her early management consultation and development work, compiled the data shown in Table 4-7, relating theory and practice. When postulating his behavioral perspectives, Maslow often stated that his theory might serve as the basis for understanding and building motivation strategies. There is little doubt that his work has stimulated the burgeoning of "motivation theories" over the past 30 years. In addition, the need hierarchy model has had great impact on organization structure, communication plans, authority, perspectives, consistent policies, and management and supervisory styles.

Managers have found Maslow's theory extremely meaningful primarily because it clearly conceptualizes their role responsibilities vis-à-vis employee motivation. The role of the manager is to create conditions of work and environment that satisfy employee needs, meeting both deficiency needs (e.g., physiological, safety, and belongingness needs) and growth needs (e.g., esteem and self-actualizing). "Failure to provide such a climate would logically lead to increased employee frustration, poorer performance, lower job satisfaction, and increased withdrawal from work activities."[23]

Vogt, in her work diagnosing organizations (climate surveys), created a checklist aimed at determining corporate motivational policies and proce-

MASLOW'S CHARACTERISTICS OF SELF-ACTUALIZATION

HONESTY

Honesty to be your feelings; to trust your feelings of humor, of anger, of love, in interpersonal relations

1. *Sense of humor:* These people have experiences that elicit a smile more usually than a laugh, that are intrinsic to the situation rather than added to it, that are spontaneous rather than planned, and that very often can never be repeated.
2. *Social interest:* They have for human beings in general a deep feeling of identification, sympathy, and affection in spite of occasional anger, impatience, or disgust.
3. *Love:* They are capable of more fusion, greater love, more perfect identification, more obliteration of the ego boundaries.

AWARENESS

Awareness of inner rightness, of nature, of the peak experiences of life

1. *Efficient perception:* They live more in the real world of nature than in the man-made mass of concepts, abstractions, expectations, beliefs, and stereotypes that most people confuse with the world.
2. *Freshness of appreciation:* They have the wonderful capacity to appreciate again and again, freshly and naively, the basic goods of life, with awe, wonder and even ecstasy.
3. *The peak experience:* The oceanic feeling; feelings of limitless horizons opening up to the vision, the feeling of being simultaneously more powerful and more helpless than one ever was before, the feeling of great ecstasy and wonder and awe, the loss of placing in time and space with, finally, the conviction that something extremely important and valuable had happened.
4. *Ethical awareness:* Strongly ethical, they have definite moral standards. Their notions of right and wrong are often not the conventional ones; they are fixed on ends rather than means.

FREEDOM

Freedom to withdraw or be detached, to be creative, to be spontaneous

1. *Detachment:* The need for privacy. They positively like solitude and privacy. It is often possible for them to remain above the battle, to remain unruffled, undisturbed.
2. *Creativeness:* A special kind of creativeness or originality or inventiveness that seems rather akin to the naive and universal creativeness of unspoiled children.
3. *Spontaneity:* Their behavior is marked by simplicity and naturalness, and by lack of artificiality or straining for effect.

TRUST

To trust in one's mission in life; to trust one's self in spite of outside influences; to trust others' nature

1. *Life mission:* These individuals customarily have some mission in life, some task to fulfill, some problem outside themselves that enlists much of their energies.
2. *Autonomy:* Independence of culture and environment; they are dependent for their own development and continued growth on their own potentialities and latent resources.
3. *Acceptance:* They can take the frailties, sins, weaknesses, and evils of human nature in the same unquestioning spirit with which one accepts the characteristics of nature.

Notes from Shostrom, E.L., producer and director: Maslow and self-actualization, Santa Ana, Calif., 1967, Psychological Films. (Film.)

TABLE 4-7

Work world applications of Maslow's need hierarchy theory of motivation

Maslow's need	Work world: examples and comments
PHYSIOLOGICAL NEEDS	Mainly satisfied through money
SAFETY NEEDS	There tend to be three categories of safety needs in work settings: 1. Physical safety; freedom from danger (job safety) 2. Emotional/human safety; freedom from threat, unemployment discrimination, favoritism; fair and consistent management 3. Job and financial security; tenure, savings accounts, insurance, recourse procedures
BELONGINGNESS AND LOVE NEEDS	Contacts with fellow employees, management persons, union representatives, and friends within the context of work—not just non-work activities *If management thwarts these needs, the person and/or an entire work force may become resistant, uncooperative, and antagonistic. It is the lack of fulfillment options at this need level that most often leads to massive unrest, strikes, and unionization efforts and activities.*
ESTEEM NEEDS	Ongoing praise for work, new responsibilities, added authority, maximum amount of control, one's own job actions, job titles, awards, status symbols, free time *Although innovations have taken place, there are relatively few opportunities for low-level (unskilled) employees to have these needs satisfied.*
SELF-ACTUALIZATION NEEDS	The experience of having one's personal autonomy and one's value to the company or organization be congruent; the person will usually enjoy the work, can continue to grow and work to the full extent of new or existing capabilities, and makes an important contribution to the organization. *There are limited opportunities at any corporate level for self-actualizing experiences.*

dures. A copy of the checklist is included on p. 128. As one can see, the first 3 criteria relate to physiological needs; the next 13 items relate to safety needs; the next 7, to belongingness needs; the next 12, to esteem needs; and the last 3, to self-actualizing needs.

A digression

Frederick Herzberg et al.,[6] building upon the groundwork laid by Maslow, developed the motivational-maintenance theory of motivation. Basically, this model states that there are elements in the work context that have to be present to maintain a state of "no dissatisfaction"; these he calls hygiene factors. They are primarily extrinsic to the job itself, and their absence causes high degrees of employee dissatisfaction. Examples of maintenance or hygiene factors are the first 23 items on the "Assessing Your

ASSESSING YOUR ORGANIZATION'S MANAGEMENT PRACTICES

Please check each item listed below for which your company has developed a formalized (written or verbalized) policy, procedure, or practice.

_____ Compensation procedures
_____ Adequate compensation as perceived by hourly employees
_____ Adequate compensation as perceived by salaried employees
_____ Criteria for job security
_____ Cleanliness
_____ Job safety standards
_____ Policy manual
_____ Fair treatment statement (within departments)
_____ Employee handbook
_____ Consistent policies (within departments)
_____ Performance appraisal system
_____ Seniority statements
_____ Antidiscrimination policies
_____ Insurance (life, health, dental) packages
_____ Savings/loans options
_____ Outlined procedures for employee recourse
_____ Teamwork opportunities
_____ Regularly scheduled meetings with immediate superior
_____ Regularly scheduled meetings with top management person(s)
_____ Access to immediate superior's superior
_____ Employee meetings
_____ Company-sponsored informal/social activities
_____ Specified breaks and mealtimes
_____ Job titles
_____ Formal recognition programs
_____ Recognition statements (from superior downward)
_____ Free time (flexibility)
_____ Promotions
_____ Additional job responsibilities
_____ Education, training, development
_____ Personal autonomy in the job task
_____ Office/desk/room space
_____ Awards for specific contributions to company productivity and/or goal achievement
_____ Recognition for service in behalf of the company
_____ Recognition for person in terms of the job responsibilities being fulfilled
_____ Corporate mission statement
_____ Company-society relationship
_____ Personal and professional growth

Source: Vogt, J.F, Supportive Management/Educational Services (SMES), Ltd., 1980.

TABLE 4-8

A graphic comparison of motivational theory constructs
of Maslow and Herzberg

Maslow's need hierarchy	Selected variables	Herzberg's motivation-maintenance model
Self-actualization	Achievement Work itself Responsibility Growth	Motivational
Esteem	Advancement Recognition Status	
Belongingness Safety	Interpersonal relationships Technical supervision Company policy and administration Job security Working conditions	Maintenance or hygiene
Physiological	{Salary	

Organization's Management Practices" checklist. Herzberg et al. also indicated that there were components within the job itself (intrinsic), and that it is these elements that are the motivators (or satisfiers). The last 15 items on the previous checklist are examples of motivational factors. Table 4-8 is provided to clarify the conceptual relationship between Maslow and Herzberg's theories. Herzberg's theory is quite popular because its terminology is work oriented and provides a simplistic model that can readily be translated into concrete activities and actions. However, it has been highly criticized as simplistic, inadequately defining job satisfaction-dissatisfaction and ignoring the importance of various job factors.

Back to Maslow

Maslow's theory has spawned an enormous amount of research, the most interesting outcome of which is that although there is minimal support for his theory of motivation, hundreds of research efforts have been carried out that *describe* corporate-organizational work life in terms of that theory. For the most part, this generalized statement is not surprising. Maslow first espoused his work as a personality theory, a way of understanding human beings and their needs; it was not intended to be a model from which specific conclusions might be drawn. It was seen, however, as so relevant, so "right" during the humanistic movement in the business world (1960s) that it was quickly espoused as a theory of motivation. Unfortunately it does not have predictive qualities—and the central goal of motivational theories is that they allow prediction. Maslow's theory, however, continues to provide one of the most meaningful ways of conceptualizing all the research findings about "people at work."

Further, it is Maslow's model (with Herzberg's additions) that has drawn our attention to *retention*. It is imperative that we recognize that motivation and retention are two separate and distinct processes *and* managerial functions. They require *different* planning and different strategies because their goals are different. It is also true that motivation and retention are intimately related for the human being—the nurse. Management must consider both goals and their "fit" in the pursuit of organizational well-being. Maslow's theory also implies self-awareness: introspection and retrospection. What are my needs and how are they (or are they not) being met? Both motivation and retention, from this theoretical posture, are equally interdependent on (a) the individual taking responsibility for knowing self and "seeking after," and (b) managerial action taking. Maslow's theory supports *nobility in the work place* —of the person, the manager, and the corporate effort.

The "cork-top (bottleneck) theory" of nurse retention

A bottleneck is a place or stage in a process at which progress is impeded. Although this chapter's primary focus is motivation, we are presenting here one theory for explaining factors affecting nurse retention. Our theory builds from Maslow's constructs regarding human needs. Picture, if you will, the cork from a bottle of champagne (see Fig. 4-5). Starting at the bottom, the cork is quite narrow; it then rounds out, giving way to its smallest diameter; the top portion spills out from itself almost in a mushroom fashion, and its very top is a slightly rounded protrusion. Starting again at the nadir, one can fit Maslow's hierarchy of needs theory quite well in terms of nurse retention. First, nurses must have their physiological needs met, and the key issue is money. As we see today's nurses, the opportunities to expand financially are greatly constricted. Given that it is upon this base that the cork fulfills its "retention" duties, it follows that this narrow "beginning" is a place to focus efforts. The next needs category, safety, has expanded according to our cork theory. Nurses have achieved rather significant personal security and safety in terms of the work place, job security, benefits, and to some extent freedom from discrimination, threat, and favoritism. It is important to note that the cork just begins to widen at this last point, indicating that management has a way to go here. Belonging and love needs follow; on the cork they begin to manifest themselves just as the cork begins to narrow. Still nurses have a great many opportunities (both formal and informal, structured and unstructured) to interact within the work setting. It is important to note, however, that the elements of corporate policy and administration—important to the belonging needs—occur at the onset of the "narrows." Esteem needs follow. They com-

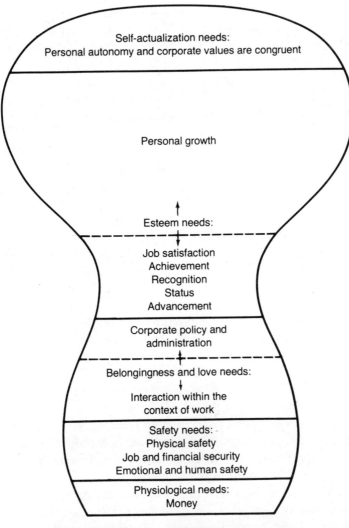

FIG. 4-5

The cork top (bottleneck) in retaining nurses. Cork top design: Korbel Champagne Cellars. (Vogt, Thames, Velthouse, Cox.)

prise the major bottleneck in management's efforts to retain nurses. Nurses receive very little job satisfaction, experience little real achievement, get little recognition, are accorded little status, and have few ways to advance other than by becoming managers. There is another form of esteem needs, those centered on the self; that is, the self must instigate satisfaction mechanisms or personal growth. Nurses have great latitude to grow personally and psychologically. They grow from the job experience, from organizational activities, from stress, from crisis, from others. They are often encouraged and helped to grow. If we look at our cork for a moment, it is interesting to note that the greatest motivational source for nurses in the work place is within self. Questions: Is this acceptable? Is the space too large? Is it fair that management's responsibilities appear so much smaller than the nurse's? Is it not time nurses come to grips with the concept of self-fulfillment, in terms of their strengths and limitations, roles and responsibilities, and power/control over their own future and joys? The final need is that of self-actualization: the process of becoming. The cork top is flat, but broad; self-actualization is all-encompassing in terms of life. The cork top holds the cork together. Again nurses are limited in their opportunities to become self-actualized because these conditions require a deeply rooted commitment to the interdependence of person-professional and the organization. This relationship very seldom exists between the two entities in today's world of health care.

It is important to point out here that nurses, according to this model, have an overwhelming opportunity to fulfill their intrinsic needs (motivators). They have not, however, secured the extrinsic maintainers—from adequate and appropriate financial remuneration to job satisfaction, achievement, and recognition. It is one of the few professions that can boast of this "reversal" from the normative conditions of work life. Nurses are motivated, but not maintained.

The implications for both hospital management and individuals are clear:

1. Recognize the "bottleneck" concept in terms of limiting accessibility to the "champagne": free flowing and yet self-limited by the size of the opened bottleneck allowing a healthy pouring out of resources.
2. Help nurses to understand the sources of constraint that so often limit their contributions. Help them to understand the sources of freedom that so often elude their perceptions.
3. Focus on those areas where the limits are excessively confining.
4. Remove the cork top. Promote interaction between the "bubbly" and the thirster, between the important resources (nurses) and their world: the hospital, the patients, the administration, their peers.

A theory is intended to help conceptualize information, to bring data into perspective. The cork-top theory of retention presented here makes a contribution to that end. We encourage our readers to consider it, expand it, alter it, use it, and/or toss it.

PROCESS AND CONTENT THEORIES OF MOTIVATION

Motivation theories have undergone significant evolution during the past 45 years. This evolution can now be looked at in retrospect and clarified according to the *focus* of the theories' efforts and intentions. One method of viewing this focus in the last few years has been to distinguish theories based on the terms process and content.

Content theories

The focus here is on those factors (needs/motives and incentives) within the person that energize, direct, sustain, stop, and start behavior. Content theories focus on inward elements that *cause* behavior. Needs or motives are direct causes of behavior (e.g., the needs for food, job security, recognition). Incentives are indirect causes of behavior in that they are external to the individual, but associated with specific needs (e.g., a promotion is an incentive related to the self-esteem need). The content theories identify *what* motivates. Most often quoted and researched content theories of motivation are Maslow's need hierarchy, Herzberg's motivational-maintenance theory, Mc-Clelland's achievement motivation, and Alderfer's ERG theory. They have all achieved well-deserved status by offering applications to the personal, managerial, and organizational responsibilities for motivation. Content theorists' major contributions have centered on job satisfaction; their efforts have led them to develop the concept of *job enrichment*.

Process theories

Process theories describe and analyze *how* behavior is energized, directed, sustained, stopped, and started. A key element has to do with individual choice: specifically, why do people choose certain behaviors to accomplish work tasks and objectives? The more current and complex process theories especially focus on two major components: perceptions (and/or expectations) and learning (the person's ability to grow, develop, change, take on new technical capabilities). Process theories tend to focus less on the internal structure of persons and more on the *external forces* impacting on the person—such as the environment within which the individual works. Major process theories include equity theory, expectancy theory, and the Porter-Lawler dynamic theory of motivation. Work-related applications of these theories have afforded major strides in affecting human behavior. Specifically, work world process theorists have focused on pay, goal setting, decision making, and leadership. It was the study of leadership that launched Kurt Lewin's work in the 1930s—the "beginning"—and it is the study of leadership and the manager that is currently consuming the energies of process theorists as they postulate vis-à-vis work.

The section in this chapter entitled "Practical Applications" more fully expands on several contributions from both process and content theories of motivation. It is noteworthy that in the last few decades, our knowledge of human behavior has mushroomed; we are indebted to those who have participated in this activity. The process and content distinction is a helpful tool. The applications to the work setting are becoming more and more prolific; many others will come from those of you reading this book.

THE MOTIVATIONAL RELATIONSHIP REVISITED: EMPLOYEE–MANAGER–ORGANIZATION

The process of motivation in the world of work is not the responsibility of the individual alone, the manager alone, or the organization alone. It is an interdependent matter. Witness this definition of motivating: *"the process of moving oneself and others to work toward attainment of individual and organizational objectives."* [14] Clearly there is a duality of responsibility: the individual and the organization. Personal activities and awareness combined with organizational policies and atmosphere directly affect motivation. Perhaps equally important to this duality is the role of the manager: the *linking pin* in the motivational process. No matter what one's hierarchical level in the organization, the manager is the identified responsible person. This manager role at all organizational levels is therefore the most *behaviorally* significant to motivating factors—be they individual or organizational. If we are concerned with staff nurses, we must consider the staff nurse's own view of self and commitment to motivation, and we must consider the hospital's policies, its administration's attitudes, and nursing's environment; but most importantly, we must consider the actions, roles, and responsibilities of the staff nurse's *direct* manager or supervisor (most often the head nurse). It is important as well to note that the head nurse must have organizational support (see the discussion of process theories of motivation in the previous section of this chapter) to fulfill the joint obligation of goal attainment. Research indicates that if the head nurse, as supervisor, is perceived as providing managerial support, the *group* of staff nurses directly subordinate to him or her will demonstrate maximum effort toward the achievement of the task. [21]

Two significant research findings support our contention regarding the importance of the head nurse (direct supervisor) in the motivational process:

1. *People work better when they have input into the decision-making process.* More fully discussed in Chapter 3, the contributions of participative management precepts, group dynamics, and communications theory have demonstrated the validity of this finding. It is important to note that providing input is defined as information giving, opinion and attitude giving, data-gathering, influencing, and/or actually decision-making responsibilities. The types of input are not nearly as crucial as the fact that input is sincerely sought and utilized. An implication for the head nurse is then to involve staff nurses actively in decision making according to (a) his or her comfort levels for including others in a particular decision area and (b) staff nurses' demonstrated wishes and capabilities.

2. *People produce at consistently higher levels—and continue an upward climb—when their goals are congruent with the organization's missions and objectives.* They in fact are becoming more self-actualized. It is imperative that the head nurse recognize this relationship and work to define the ways in which each staff nurse's contributions to the work place match the organization's needs according to its goals. The head nurse must *verbalize* this relationship on an ongoing basis to the staff nurse as well as to immediate superiors. Second, the head nurse needs to be aware that "becoming" is just as important as "getting there." True self-actualization is a process far more than an accomplishment. Head nurses must recognize the contributions staff nurses make daily as a "matter of routine" as directly contributing to the "routine" functions of the organization. In this way, staff nurses offer themselves to the highest of causes on a daily basis. Again both general and specific verbal recognition of this point to subordinates and superiors must become a consistent activity and major responsibility for head nurses. Historically, nurses have been hospital oriented. In recent years their focus has been on themselves within the framework of personal autonomy. It is of merit to realize that through self-actualization, a person's effort and well-being as well as the organization's effort and well-being can bring about a mutuality of achievement.

Motivation as a system of exchange

Recognizing the impact on motivation of this employee-organization interdependency can lead to interpreting motivation as a system of exchange.* Two assumptions are basic to a motivational theory of exchange. First, each party enters the relationship because each has something to gain that the other has to offer. This makes the exchange concept one that rests on an equality of contribution. The second assumption has to do with a characteristic of the relationship, that is, that an equitable exchange can be maintained. It is the combination of these two assumptions that pertains to *retaining* and *motivating* staff nurses in health care settings. An example of the kinds of contributions that can be exchanged in the employee-organization relationship is presented in Table 4-9.

Although each entity may recognize the equity factor in the relationship, each may not agree on what is equal. The key in some ways is balance. The more this balance is achieved, through open communications and honest concern for the other (optimal exchange), the higher the motivation of each individual. On the other hand, the more the balance is achieved through power, manipulation, and/or coercion, the greater the likelihood there will be an

---

*The discussions of Homans,[7] Steers and Porter,[20] and Williams[24] regarding the concepts of exchange have been most helpful to the authors on this point.

TABLE 4-9

Possible contributions in the employee-organization exchange

Organizational contributions to fulfilling employee needs	Employee contributions to fulfilling organization needs
Financial compensation	Support of goals
Safe working conditions	Dependability
Job security	Loyalty
Fair treatment	Cooperation
Social relationships	Problem-solving behavior
Status and power	Initiative
Responsibility	Creativity
Growth opportunities	Productivity

Based on data from Williams, J. Clifton: Human Behavior in Organizations, Cincinnati, Ohio, 1978, South Western Publishing Co., pp. 119-120. The information also tracks Maslow's hierarchy of needs theory.

increase in employee turnover. *Balancing*—working toward mutually satisfy-ing the needs of two or more parties—is the crux of an exchange theory of motivation.

Balancing must go beyond the exchange of a day's work for a day's pay if motivation is to be truly achieved. It must focus on those factors that are im-portant to each *specific* organization-employee circumstance. What are appro-priate factors for hospital A may or may not be important in hospital B. Thus each environment must be separately and uniquely considered. In the ex-change theory context this is especially important because it is not merely the *outcomes* that result, but the *process* of *how* the outcomes are reached, that affect motivation. The implications of the theory of exchange for health care organizations are twofold:

1. Each health care organization must *identify* those specific exchange items that fit its operations, circumstances, policies, leaders, and em-ployees.
2. Therefore, each must *develop* a process for exchange, that is, for ful-filling individual and organization needs. This process must be char-acterized by openness, healthy communications, respect, and a true concern for meeting the others' needs.

The exchange theory of motivation discards the notion of cookbook solu-tions; there are none in the sense of "if an organization does X, then its em-ployees will be Y or Z." The following section, "Practical Applications," will focus on one part of the exchange process: assessment. Chapter 8 will expand the process even further. It is imperative to the success of the balancing pro-cess that each participant in the process have a sound knowledge of relevant motivation theories and research findings. The greater the knowledge base, the more likely a sound exchange *system,* as well as descriptive components of the exchange, will be lasting and appropriate. It is important to point out that we are advocating a systemwide process here, one component of which probably will include employee-supervisor dialogue and applications. The system provides the environment for quality or nonquality interactions. According to research by Rensis Likert, the interaction, the styles and outcomes, and the relationships occurring at the very top of an organization are mirrored throughout that organization at each and every level of corporate operation and individual activity. The systemwide process will therefore be a model for all focused interactions.

There are *foundation factors* in the exchange system. In other words, there are certain elements that are "given"—that are not to be "agreed on." These are factors that define the conditions necessary for a mutually appropriate exchange to occur. On the organization-management side, these foundation factors include relating to employees in ways that enhance their self-worth, dignity, and respect; treating employees fairly; and providing a safe work place. Nothing should be expected in return for these actions. Employees, on the other hand, must work toward the accomplishment of corporate missions especially in terms of their job responsibilities. These foundations are central to the employee-organizational relationship. Additionally, the more genuine and nonmanipulative the attempts to meet the other's needs, the greater the trusting qualities of the relationship. The greater the trust, the more likely the exchange will lead to high levels of organization and employee well-being. It is also true that this foundation paves the way for adjustments, a fact of life in today's world.

The exchange theory of motivation described here is in many ways a framework for this book on retention. It is also a kind of justification for the living-working relationship. It is a "tight" theory that has ties with the world in such areas as values, religion, and *raisons d'être* for us all.

PRACTICAL APPLICATIONS

This section is intended to give our readers some places to start with regard to motivation. First, those whose responsibilities are to deal effectively with motivation must have a sound knowledge base. Included below is a design for a 3-day workshop to build this foundation. Another component necessary to explore is whether the behaviors that are of concern are *motivation* related or *performance* related. Questions for making this determination are presented. Job enrichment has long been a recognized strategy for motivating individuals; presented here are some questions that might be used by supervisors to identify sources of job enhancement for each employee. Finally, this section contains a questionnaire that can be utilized to determine the degree to which a particular job actually fulfills a person's needs; it allows the supervisor to determine motivational levels being tapped by the current work situation. The instrument can also be used to identify organizational patterns that may exist. Further, the reader is urged to refer back to the survey form entitled, "Assessing Your Organization's Management Practices" (p. 128) for an excellent checklist of organizational responsibilities in the motivation process. Before elaborating on each of these applications, a word of caution and a word of help are in order. Issues related to motivation do not occur in a vacuum; they occur in relation to the big picture. It is this larger consideration that we address in Chapter 8, where we examine the "whole" in terms of planned change and/or organizational development. It is therefore necessary to inform the reader that undertaking any of the activities presented here will probably create a system of imbalance causing stress within the organization. An organization must change to reduce the staying power of continuously unresolved stress or high degrees of dysfunctional stress. The word of caution is do *not* undertake any of these activities unless the organization and its membership are willing to change, and preferably unless these activities are seen as part of a broader plan of organizational change. The resulting consequences of such action taking may in the long run be far greater than doing nothing. Chapter 8 not only expands on those concepts but also provides the basics for a more broadly based organizational development plan. Also, because the crux and starting points for such endeavors are data-gathering activities, guidelines for utilizing assessment questionnaires are more carefully explored in Chapter 8. One other source of help for those who wish to proceed with the activities described below is the consultant. The consultant may be from another department within the institution, may be a formal internal organization consultant, or may be a professional external consultant. At any rate, seek out an objective person who can *help* to explore and design the intervention process necessary to your circumstances. Although a person with a good knowledge of motivation is important, it is far more imperative that a consultant be chosen who understands the process of personal and organizational *change*. Again, this prerequisite is further expanded upon in Chapter 8.

A 3-day workshop on motivation

The workshop design on pp. 139-141 is presented in sufficient depth for a qualified facilitator—whether internal or external to the organization—to provide a meaningful and productive learning experience. The workshop was designed by Judy Vogt with the expressed purpose of providing participants personal insights, theoretical input, and managerial-supervisory and organizational behavioral applications. The optimum group size for this workshop is 24; the more skilled the facilitator, the more diverse group membership can be. It is intended, however, to be utilized with participants from a single facility.

MOTIVATION WORKSHOP

Activities	Materials and supplies

DAY 1

A. Overview of the workshop

Agenda (optional), easel, newsprint, markers, blackboard and chalk

B. A small group activity (4 to 6 persons)
  1. Participants discuss *"specific* situations with which they are familiar having to do with motivation."
  2. Theory input on how to make statements in *proposition* form
  3. Participants make proposition statements from the experiences discussed in B,1.
  4. These statements are put on newsprint and posted; the total group then takes a "walking tour."

Newsprint, magic markers, masking tape/group

  5. Total group discussion
  6. Theory input: relationship between experience and theory

C. Brief theory input on the following general concepts related to motivation:
  1. Sustained, ongoing effort
  2. Planned or recognized activities
  3. Individual matter
  4. Motivation: productivity and life

D. Lecturette and small group discussion on expectancy theory

Chapter 4, *Retaining Professional Nurses*

  1. See "Expectancy-Valence Theory, Expanded" in this chapter.
  2. Encourage participants to relate the concepts first to themselves and *then* to their work setting.

E. Film: "Productivity and the self-fulfilling prophecy"

Film (28 min.)

  1. Self-time: What does this mean to me?
  2. Small group discussion, implications to managers-supervisors

F. Two main framework theories

Chapter 4, *Retaining Professional Nurses*
Self-assessment activities

  1. Douglas McGregor
  2. Abraham Maslow (and Herzberg)
  3. Facilitators are encouraged to utilize self-assessment activities as well as lecture and small-group discussion.

G. Homework: two articles (these or others as appropriate)

"One More Time, How Do You Motivate Employees" (Frederick Herzberg). "Misconceptions About Motivation" (Howard Smith, Training/HRD, March 1979)

H. Evaluation: process and content of the day; self, small group, total group; informal

Continued.

MOTIVATION WORKSHOP—cont'd

Activities	Materials and supplies
DAY 2	
A. Introduction: informal total group discussion Plan for the day, yesterday (Day 1) in retrospect, reactions to the homework assignments	
B. Theory input and small group discussion of Porter-Lawler model (expectancy theory)	Chapter 4, *Retaining Professional Nurses*
C. The job and motivation—brief theory input	
1. Focus on the need for the supervisor to know how employees see their job.	
2. Small groups generate possible assessment questions that may be utilized by supervisors to assess employees' perceptions about their jobs.	Paper and pencil/group
3. Caution: Use assessment only if action taking will follow.	
4. Small groups share their questions; these are later typed, reproduced, and distributed to participants	
D. Report: Jay Hall study (1978); attention should be drawn to the interrelatedness of the five variables as well as to the findings. This should be in lecture form with free-flowing questions and answers.	Jay Hall research report or notes (1978 study of 16,000 managers and supervisors) for lecture purpose only
E. Each participant is given a copy of the Farson article on praise to read and then encouraged to reflect on it; adequate and active small group dialogue is imperative after reading this article. Personal implications are numerous.	"Praise Reappraised" (Richard Farson)
F. Self-time: Each participant reviews the content portion of the workshop and draws own conclusions on:	
1. Job activities	
2. Personal style	
G. Homework: "What does all of this mean for our organization?" Think about it.	
H. More formal evaluation of:	An evaluation form
1. Content features	
2. Activities	
3. Facilitator(s)	
DAY 3	
A. Small work groups are formed, which will be fixed for the day and may have "after-workshop" life.	Papers, pencils, paper clips, tape, newsprint, felt markers (various colors), masking tape
B. Groups are asked to begin exploring their organization in terms of issues related to motivation. This information is shared. Adequate dialogue and conflict resolution time (and perhaps activities) must be allowed. Representatives of each group meet to determine "action steps(s)." The importance here is to follow up, not to design an entire "plan."	

MOTIVATION WORKSHOP—cont'd

Activities	Materials and supplies

DAY 3—cont'd

C. The total group then chooses two departments or groups or levels within the organization to focus on—probably those where motivation issues (not performance issues) are most crucial. The same process (see B above) is utilized for each. Groups may be realigned according to relevant similar criteria in order to work on group-specific issues if appropriate.

  Facilitators may want to supply various theory or diagnostic materials to facilitate the process. *All process issues must be worked on before proceeding.*

D. The workshop concludes with an overview of the concepts presented—those related to the topic matter (motivation) as well as the process (group issues and work-oriented issues).

Assessment questions: a matter of motivation or performance

Often organizations are unclear about whether an employee's behaviors are motivation related or performance related. Let us distinguish between the two here.* First, motivation concerns occur when there is a discrepancy between what is expected and what actually results; this discrepancy must be due to a lack of effort on the employee's part as well to be classified as motivational. Second, performance concerns occur when an employee's behavior does not measure up to expectations. Performance problems may or may not be the result of low motivation. It is highly likely, however, that such problems arise out of one or more other problems. The following questions must be asked by each supervisor before attributing poor performance to low motivation:

- Have I adequately clarified to the employee what is expected of him or her? *(communication)*
- Do I know whether the employee has the mental or physical capabilities to perform the job? *(ability)*
- Have I adequately prepared the employee for the job requirements? *(training)*
- Have I created the proper environment and are the proper conditions in place to allow the person to do the job? *(opportunity)*

*Much of this discussion was generated from the perspectives of J. Williams in his book, *Human Behavior in Organizations*.[24] See specifically "How to Analyze a Motivation Problem," p. 135.

Assessing the job: searching for ways to enrich work

Supervisors (whether they are presidents, directors, managers, or head nurses) can greatly enhance the quality of work a subordinate contributes by learning how that employee experiences his or her job. After gleaning this information, the supervisor can work collaboratively with the individual and the environment to improve job features and activities. The supervisor also gathers data that afford a big picture and allow the opportunity to recognize how the structure of work or job descriptions fit group and individual goals and needs. Though both of these tasks are time consuming and require highly developed analysis, organizing, and planning skills, the rewards in terms of human motivation in behalf of the job are often enormous.

The following list of questions presents possible choices; or make up your own. Give consideration to the actual format of the survey questions (written or verbal), time factor, and data feedback methods. Remember, do not ask a question on which you do not intend to take action.

POSSIBLE JOB EVALUATION QUESTIONS

What do you like best about your job?

What do you like least about your job?

In your opinion, what job duties do you perform best?

What job duties do you feel you need to improve on?

Are there any job duties or responsibilities that you would like clarified?

In the past 90 days, what *three* things have happened that caused you to feel particularly bad about your job?

In the past 90 days, what *three* things have happened that caused you to feel particularly good about your job?

Would you prefer a different position at _____? If so, which one, and why?

What are your personal goals for the next 2 years? How does your job help you achieve these goals?

Is there any training or assistance you believe you need to perform your job more efficiently?

What is the most challenging thing you have done in your present job?

What is the thing you find most tedious in your job?

What would make your job easier and more satisfying (surroundings, equipment, interactions with others, supervisor, etc.)?

Do you feel your job requires more or fewer responsibilities? Explain.

If given the opportunity, how would you change your job?

Is your job a source of reward for you? If yes, how? If yes or no, discuss.

Are you provided with sufficient room to grow?

If in your power, what would you change about your job?

When do you feel is your "lowest ebb" during the day?

What qualities of your job give you particular satisfaction?

Identifying motivational elements of the job: a questionnaire

Persons relate to their jobs individually according to their motivation needs. Determining the motivational needs being fulfilled by the job in conjunction with how important the job is to an employee is a first step in determining motivation-related issues. The questionnaire on p. 144 not only focuses on specific needs but also can be categorized according to Maslow's or Herzberg's need groups. Appropriate maintenance or developmental actions can then be planned for each employee or group of employees. This questionnaire can also be used on an organizationwide basis to identify any general patterns within the system; again both Maslow's and Herzberg's theories can be used as means for analyzing the data. Additionally, the broader application may identify one or two consistent strengths and/or limitations that are organization-specific tendencies.

Information gleaned from this questionnaire and the preceding questions can often pinpoint strategies for improving staff development functions (e.g., selection, training) as well as designing innovative job enrichment programs in such areas as placement (rotation and matching) and promotion (e.g., parallel career path options or the career ladder concept).

A CONCEPTUAL CONCLUSION

This chapter has examined motivation. It has drawn implications for understanding motivation as it relates to staff nurses. It has also differentiated motivation factors from retention factors. Though separate and distinct constructs, motivation and retention may in the last analysis still be affected by the same exact variable depending on the person and the circumstances. So in closing, we must reach for a new concept, a different way to explain retention in relation to motivation. Perhaps such a new perspective lies within the concept of *commitment*.

Traditionally, commitment has been related to two variables: one is performance (the motivational factor) and one is membership (the retention factor). An important question for us at this point in the book is: Why will an individual retain membership with an organization despite the absence of a myriad of key exchange factors relevant to the motivational process? Richard Scholl[18] has hypothesized four possible sources for such individual staying power: investment, reciprocity, lack of alternatives, and identification. Brief descriptions of each of these sources follow here:

- *Investment:* the degree to which continued membership is tied to future gain
- *Reciprocity:* the belief that one should help not harm those who have helped one in the past
- *Lack of alternatives:* the degree to which one's capabilities and skills

ORGANIZATIONAL MOTIVATION NEED INVENTORY

Rank each of the following 21 motivational characteristics on a scale of 1 (very little) to 7 (very high). Do this for parts A and B.

Motivational characteristics	Part A How much do I now have?	Part B How much do I want?
1. *Pay* for my job		
2. The feeling of *security* in my job		
3. *Working conditions* surrounding my job		
4. Amount of *pressure* I feel in my job		
5. Organization *policies* and the way they are administered		
6. Competence of our *management* people		
7. Chance to develop *close friendships* on the job		
8. Chance to *help others* in my job		
9. Being *informed* in my job		
10. The *recognition* I receive in my job		
11. *Prestige* of my job *inside* the organization		
12. *Prestige* of my job *outside* the organization		
13. The *authority* connected with my job		
14. Amount of *responsibility* I have		
15. The feeling of *self-esteem* in my job		
16. Participation in *setting methods and procedures* for my job		
17. Opportunity to participate in *goal setting*		
18. Feeling of *worthwhile accomplishment* I have in my job		
19. Opportunity for *personal growth and development*		
20. Opportunity for *independent thought and action* in my job		
21. *Self-fulfillment* I have in my job		

Adapted from Omni System. Used with permission.

are seen as fitting the organization of which one currently is a member
• *Identification:* the linking of one's social identity to a specific role
Any one or combination of these factors can serve as a source of commitment.

The ramifications for health care institutions vis-à-vis the retention (and motivation) of professional nurses are numerous. No longer can managers be willing to "let things ride," although Scholl's hypotheses imply just the opposite. We now know at least some factors that explain the existence of commitment despite the possibilities of numerous inequities in the employee-organization relationship. Of course we need further creative thinking and a great deal of research to substantiate these considerations. However, we already do know that *there is an explanation:* commitment too has antecedents; it does not just occur. Human beings are constantly seeking new understandings in terms of their behavior. Staff nurses are human beings. They will begin to learn why they stay and to personally examine these factors in light of their needs. Managers must work with their employees to facilitate the exploration of this process for organizations to survive and for people to retain their integrity. Health care organizations must now reexamine the element of commitment as it relates to retention and ultimately to motivation. Staying is not enough for today's health care needs, be they institutional or personal. It is highly likely that by exploring this issue of commitment more fully, health care can make meaningful strides in the retention and motivation of staff nurses. Membership and performance are intricately linked, and in the long run, it is this linkage that is of ultimate significance in the world of work and in the experiencing of life. It is a fitting exploration in which the joint efforts of employees and organizations can come together to make a difference. Commitment can serve as the rallying point for a mutual process and for a new age that defines the quality of nursing's contributions to health care.

REFERENCES AND ADDITIONAL READINGS

1. Adams, J.S.: Toward an understanding of inequity, J. Abnor. Soc. Psychol. **67**(5):422-436, Nov. 1963.
2. Boone, L.E., and Kurtz, D.L.: Principles of management, New York, 1981, Random House.
3. Duncan, W.J.: Organizational behavior, ed. 2, Boston, 1981, Houghton-Mifflin Co.
4. Gibson, J.L., Ivancevich, J.M., and Donnelly, J.H., Jr.: Organizations: behavior, structure, process, ed. 4, Plano, Tex., 1982, Business Publications, Inc.
5. Hall, C.S., and Lindsey, G.: Theories of personality, New York, 1973, John Wiley & Sons.
6. Herzberg, F., Mausner, B., and Synderman, B.: The motivation to work, New York, 1959, John Wiley & Sons.
7. Homans, G.C.: Social behavior exchange, Am. J. Sociol. **63**(6):597-606, May 1958.
8. Katz, D., and Kahn, R.: The social psychology of organizations, ed. 2, New York, 1978, John Wiley & Sons.

9. Likert, R.: The human organization: its management and value, New York, 1967, McGraw-Hill Book Co.
10. McGregor, D.: The human side of enterprise, New York, 1960, McGraw-Hill Book Co.
11. McGregor, D.: The professional manager, New York, 1967, McGraw-Hill Book Co.
12. Menlo, A.: The growing of persons: speculations, readings, and activities in the actualization of human potential. Office of Instructional Services, School of Education, The University of Michigan, Ann Arbor, 1980.
13. Menlo, A.: The University of Michigan. Formal and Informal Person-Person Interaction (1963 to Present).
14. Mescon, M., Albert, M., and Khedouri, F.: Management, New York, 1981, Harper & Row.
15. Porter, L.W., and Lawler, E.E., III: Managerial attitudes and performance, Homewood, Ill., 1968, Dorsey-Irwin.
16. Renwick, P.A., Lawler, E.E., and Psychology Today staff: What you really want from your job, Psychol. Today 11(12):53, May 1978.
17. Robinson, A.J.: McGregor's theory X–theory Y model, Ann. Hdbk. Group Facilitators, 4:121-123, 1972.
18. Scholl, R.W.: Differentiating organizational commitment from expectancy as a motivating force, Acad. Mgmt. Rev. 6(4):589-599, Oct. 1981.
19. Steers, R.: Introduction to organizational behavior, Glenview, Ill., 1981, Scott, Foresman and Co.
20. Steers, R., and Porter, L.: Motivation and work behavior, New York, 1975, McGraw-Hill Book Co.
21. Szilagyi, A.D., and Wallace, M.J.: Organizational behavior and performance, ed. 2, Santa Monica, Calif. 1980, Goodyear Publishing Co.
22. Telly, C.S., French, W.L., and Scott, W.G.: The relationship between inequity to turnover among hourly workers, Admin. Sci. Quart. 16:164-172, 1972.
23. Vroom, V.H.: Work and motivation, New York, 1964, John Wiley & Sons.
24. Williams, J.C.: Human behavior in organizations, Cincinatti, Ohio, 1978, South Western Publishing Co.

5

ONGOING PROFESSIONALIZATION

INTRODUCTION: PROFESSIONALISM AND NURSING
Unique body of knowledge and skill
Long and disciplined educational process
Commitment
Autonomy/discretionary authority
Active and cohesive professional organization
Acknowledged social worth and contribution
Self-governance

BUILDING INTO THE SYSTEM
Professional opportunities
Clinical, managerial, educational, and specialist options
Personal and interpersonal growth
Leadership training

INDIVIDUALITY AND JOB DESIGN CONSIDERATIONS
Flexible scheduling
Job redesign and job enrichment

PROGRAM DESIGN
A CONCEPTUAL CONCLUSION

INTRODUCTION: PROFESSIONALISM AND NURSING

Nursing is a profession, although it has not consistently met all of the criteria associated with professions or demonstrated the degree of dedication to occupational standards of performance that is compatible with professionalism. The premise underlying a profession has always been synonymous with a blend of individual and group growth, acceptance, and self-governance. A major impediment to the full acceptance of nursing as a profession has been that conceptually this premise has not been internalized in the beliefs, opinions, and actions of nurses themselves. Although debates on whether nursing is a true profession still ensue, the important consideration is that professionalization, which implies "giving professional character to," is what nursing is doing: nursing is in the process of becoming.

Certain criteria are utilized to determine what constitutes a profession. These criteria are here presented and discussed in an attempt to explore their fit with nursing as a profession. Nurses in the 1980s are declaring that they are professional and they want recognition, privileges, and responsibilities commensurate with this status. Professional criteria and comments on their relation to nursing follow.

Unique body of knowledge and skill

It has long been recognized that nursing needs to amass a unique body of knowledge related to nursing practice. Over the past decade there has been an increased emphasis on nursing research, especially as it relates to clinical practice. Research involves disciplined study into the effects of nursing actions that will ultimately lead to standards of practice, standards that will originate from specialists in nursing and not from administrative edicts. Sources of funds to continue this research must be identified and tapped. The American Nurses' Foundation is becoming more aggressive in soliciting money from private individuals to perpetuate the kinds of research vital to establishing a basis for nursing as a profession. This criterion is in the process of being met. Professional nursing includes but is not limited to those skills and knowledge found on p. 149.

Long and disciplined educational process

Nursing, with its three entry levels into the profession, remains in a real dilemma in health care education and preparation. Other professions (e.g., medicine, dentistry, law, education) experienced this problem early in their history before successfully adapting and changing. For example, in 1910 the Flexner Commission and Flexner report called for sweeping reform in medical education of the day, and this was accomplished. Goldmark in 1923, and Brown in 1943 were advocating changes in nursing education. The initial report and preliminary recommendation of the National Commission on

**PROFESSIONAL NURSING:
UNIQUE BODY OF KNOWLEDGE AND SKILLS**

KNOWLEDGE OF

Nursing process: assessment, planning, implementation, evaluation
Asepsis
Standards of nursing practice
Communication techniques: verbal and nonverbal communication
Interpersonal communication
Anatomy and physiology
Pathophysiology
Physical assessment: inspection, auscultation, percussion, and palpation
Diagnostic and laboratory assessment: blood work, X rays, and bacteriological studies
Principles of problem solving
Theories of behavioral psychology
Adaptation techniques
High-level wellness
Stages of death and dying
Distortion of body image

SKILLS IN

Patient assessment techniques
Interviewing techniques
Patient teaching
Patient discharge planning (including patient and significant others in plan)
Communicating effectively with patient
Identifying patient's psychological and physiological needs based on subjective and objective data
Interpreting laboratory and diagnostic data
Relating the patient's pathophysiology to normal anatomy and physiology
Problem-oriented medical recording
Family counseling

Nursing, released in 1981, concluded that the existence of three types of basic nursing education creates confusion and uncertainty in the minds of the public, employing agencies, and prospective nursing candidates as to the optimal preparation for the professional nurse. The commission further states that baccalaureate education for professional nursing practice is a desirable goal. In the early 1980s, nursing as a whole had no consensus on basic educational preparation, and in the ranks of practitioners this continues to be the number one issue dividing the profession. Nursing remains handicapped by an educational process that has been bifurcated—part collegiate and part noncollegiate. Even worse, it is stagnated by leaders, educators, and practitioners who can neither articulate the concept nor support the need for a consistent uniform educational base for entry into the practice of professional nursing.

Commitment

A hallmark of a profession is reflected in the commitment of its practitioners. Nursing includes a large share of loyal members within its ranks. Conversely, this professional quality is not consistently evident among nursing's practitioners. Professionals do not withdraw, retire early, stop work entirely, take long hiatuses, then resume. Nor do they assume other job-related activities such as sales representation for industry; these are incompatible with commitment to the practice of professional nursing.

In medicine the average working lifetime is 40 or more years. In nursing, it is approximately 20 years. This is only slightly better than any American female of high school education or beyond whose working lifetime is 19½ years. These statistics do not reflect a professional commitment; but even more astounding is the fact that the average staff nurse position in the United States experiences a 70% turnover in a 12-month period.[15] This migrancy syndrome is not compatible with professional commitment.

Nursing must have a uniform commitment toward higher level practice as evidenced by the following:

1. Intent to stay: the intent to stay as a dimension of commitment has been found to have the largest impact on turnover. This supports what others such as Price and Mueller[22] have contended, that commitment is more important than job satisfaction.
2. Concern for patients: a concern for patients (clients) manifests itself in the quality of care delivered by nursing practitioners. The degree of trust the public places in a profession rests with the individual licensed practitioner. The license obligates the nurse to practice well. It is in this way that nursing fulfills its commitment to society.

Autonomy/discretionary authority

As licensed professionals, nurses expect to display and exercise discretion in the work place. They want to participate in hospital policy decisions that affect their practice, but this seldom happens. What does happen is that nurses become resigned to *not* making a difference, which produces career stagnation and disillusionment with nursing. Nursing must (1) provide itself opportunities to develop freely, so that nurses can have the opportunity to choose, to learn, to grow; (2) have the authority to regulate the practice of its practitioners through licensure, certification, and advanced practice for the protection of the public; (3) work in cooperation and collaboration with other health care professionals; and (4) unite its multiple specialty groups in order to speak with one voice of authority.

Active and cohesive professional organization

The American Nurses' Association (ANA), the organization that purportedly speaks for all of nursing, has neither the numbers nor the cohesiveness to be a reckoning force for change. According to available statistics, slightly more than 200,000[15] or about 20% of registered nurses employed in the United States are members of ANA. Complicating the effectiveness of this professional organization even further is the existence of multiple specialty groups (somewhere between 20 and 30 in number) and of the National League for Nursing (NLN).

The responsibility of the professional organization too often is narrowly viewed as being concerned with (1) economic and general welfare, (2) legislative affairs, and (3) educational and practice issues that confront nursing. Frequently overlooked is the responsibility that the professional organization has toward (1) promoting collegiality among nursing groups and other health professions; and (2) supporting, reinforcing, collaborating with, and encouraging dialogue and good interpersonal/interprofessional relations among nursing's diverse constituencies.

The specialty nursing organizations have usually been organized to meet specific educational and affiliation needs of nurses practicing in a particular clinical area. They further blur the cohesiveness of nursing because not only do many accept members who are not registered nurses, but they do not align themselves with or recommend membership in the ANA. A positive move in recent years, however, has been the formation of the Federation of Specialty Nursing Organizations. This has allowed a mechanism to promote dialogue and cohesiveness among the various specialty groups and the ANA.

The NLN, organized primarily for educational purposes, has two types of memberships: individual and agency. Individual members may be registered nurses, practical nurses, allied health professionals, or laypersons. This mixture of professional and nonprofessional members further confuses those within and without the profession and serves to diminish the prestige associated with this organization.

Nursing needs to be able to unite the members of the profession to speak for all of nursing. It will then have a sense of its own professional worth and will display its value to physicians, administrators, legislators, the general public, and itself. It will demonstrate (1) the value of nursing care and (2) the ability of nursing to improve the practice of the profession.

Acknowledged social worth and contribution

Nursing as a profession has long enjoyed strong public support and admiration. Largely based on the public's perception of nursing as a "soft" discipline with images of Florence Nightengale providing care to the sick, this has further confounded the road to professionalization of nursing. The public likes what it thinks nursing is, and has failed to understand how it has changed and how it must change to be a true profession. Nursing has begun to articulate its cause more clearly and effectively to the public, and to initiate more interaction with consumer groups and interdisciplinary bodies. It is timely and essential that nursing seek public participation and active support in its efforts to professionalize.

In addition to the criteria that nursing must meet to be called professional, individual nurses must demand professionalism of each and every practitioner.

An uninformed public cannot be expected to make a reasonable judgment concerning what nursing is, its value to patient care, and its worth as a profession. Considering all health care practicing professions, nursing alone has the numbers of clinically competent practitioners to effect a difference in health care as we know it today. However, numbers are not enough. Without unity and consistent growth, nurses and nursing will too often be relegated to the bottom rung in the hospital organizational hierarchy, and there they will stay—divided, fragmented, bitter, and disillusioned.

Self-governance

Nursing is often characterized as a paraprofession caught in an ambiguous organizational position between hospital administration and medical staff. The uniquely distinguishing characteristic of professions is the socially sanctioned right to control their own work and members. Nursing control does exist and is recognized at lower levels (e.g., patient care units), but less so at the organizational level (e.g., administrative and board of trustees meetings). Hospital administration and medical staff continue to tolerate nursing as a "sorority," a necessary evil; but they deny these professionals, worthy to be called colleagues, a full partnership in the provision of health care. To assist nurses in ongoing professionalization and to provide opportunities for growth, development, and maturation of their knowledge and skills, some areas of clinical, managerial, and administrative behavior must be recognized, categorized, and dealt with effectively.

Much of the remainder of this chapter is devoted to separate examination of topics relevant to growth and professionalization. The chapter concludes with program design—an overview of crucial considerations, processes, and methodologies when planning ongoing professionalism opportunities for nursing—and a conceptual conclusion.

BUILDING INTO THE SYSTEM

Are there professional opportunities for nurses? Is nursing only "women's work"? Is nursing perceived as a successful occupation? Can the individual nurse's role in nursing be meaningful to self? Does society really value nursing? If one pauses to contemplate the answers to these questions, many ideas for professional development emerge. A profession that values excellence in itself will continue to develop. Nursing has the responsibility to continue to find ways in which excellence is promoted and nurtured. The commitment to ongoing professionalism is manifest by having growth and development options built into the system's structure rather than as appendixes or budgetary extensions. Specifically, nursing has a responsibility to incorporate professional opportunities; clinical, managerial, educational, and specialist options; personal and interpersonal growth; and leadership training.

Professional opportunities

Physical and emotional health. A shortcoming of many hospitals as they try to attract and retain nurses is a lack of focus on the personal life, goals, aspirations, and values of the individual nurse. Hospital and nursing administrations too often concentrate on the professional life of employees to the exclusion of the life of the nurse outside the hospital. Tied very closely with the need to balance personal needs and professional requirements is the need for activities to improve the physical and mental well-being of employees working in an emotionally charged, stressful environment. Many hospitals have an active, proactive employee health department offering prophylaxis, health counseling, and assessment facilities. Some hospitals now provide recreational activities: team sports, trips, classes, and facilities to assist the employee in meeting some of these personal needs. Other hospitals have tennis courts, jogging tracks, and swimming pools. This concept needs to be further developed and made more consistent throughout the health care industry. To assist the employee further in attaining and maintaining a state of wellness, good employee health-screening policies, practices, and facilities must be developed. An employer who recognizes and deems important the employee's emotional health needs will make provisions for the personal growth of the employee during his or her work life as well as provide basic management practices that recognize mental and emotional health needs in the work area.

Professional growth. As we demand more and more from nurses with respect to patient care, application of technological innovations, increased specialization, and management of personnel, it is imperative that nurses be asked about their expectations, motivations, needs, goals, ideas, and recommendations. Primary nursing as a mode of delivering nursing care has been revived in recent years and is enjoying tremendous popularity in hospitals today as nurses make the self-conscious declaration that patient care is the nurse's territory. Primary nursing is really more a philosophy than a way of delivering care. At last, patients know who is responsible and accountable for the outcomes of their care and the nurse has responsibility and authority for a group of patients that is commensurate with the role for which he or she was prepared.

Joint practice committees are being established in hospitals so that nurses and physicians can work together in the development of standards for patient care. This climate fosters collegiality and understanding of the role, value, and contribution of each discipline. Collaborative relationships among schools of nursing faculties who are advancing the practice through research, as well as clinical practice settings where expert clinicians work as partners to improve nursing care, are enhancing professional growth for nurses in both education and service (e.g., The Rush-Presbyterian Medical Center Project in Chicago). Significant numbers of nurses are seeking certification for professional achievement in specific practice arenas, such as those offered through the ANA and other specialty nursing groups. This will afford nurses the opportunity to be recognized for clinical excellence individually and collectively. Enlightened employers are also recognizing this achievement with financial remuneration.

Every day in hospitals, a significant number of nurses reveal a desire and need for professional growth opportunities through subtle and direct appeals. It is indicated in staff meetings, in discussions with peers and supervisors, by requests to attend outside workshops and seminars, and by requests for educational or in-service programs provided within the hospitals. Some commonly accepted ways of meeting these needs are listed on p. 155.

Opportunity to learn new skills. Nursing administration has an obligation to its employees to provide opportunities to learn new skills. This can be accomplished in a variety of ways but is best facilitated by a progressive, innovative staff development department. A system must be in place that allows identification of nurses desiring to learn new skills. Identification may occur either by a formal request to transfer from one nursing unit to another or by a request for enrollment in educational sessions provided by the nursing education department. Most frequently, nursing's requests for specific educational programs within the hospital are made by staff via administrative staff to the nursing education department, where the programs are planned, speakers or instructors are secured, and the program is scheduled. A few examples of programs that provide nurses the knowledge and skills to facilitate movement into a new clinical area are (1) coronary care module, (2) critical care module, (3) trauma nursing series, (4) hemodynamic monitoring workshop, (5) postgraduate operating room nursing course, and (6) obstetrical nursing course.

The trend in nursing in the past 20 years has been to specialize and remain in that specialty throughout the nursing career. Recent moves, however, based on the Japanese industrial model (and job rotation/enrichment constructs), have been instituted that allow nurses to be trained in more than one specialty, thereby offering more career options and opportunities for in-

---

PROFESSIONAL GROWTH POSSIBILITIES

OPPORTUNITIES FOR CONTINUING EDUCATION

Within the institution: conferences, classes to upgrade knowledge and skills or prepare a nurse for practice in a new clinical area

Outside the institution (financial and time compensation): workshops, seminars, national nursing conferences, and specialty meetings

IN-SERVICE EDUCATION

New products, equipment, techniques (provided by education instructors and manufacturers' representatives)

OPPORTUNITY TO CONTINUE FORMAL EDUCATION

University setting: tuition reimbursement programs

PARTICIPATION ON COMMITTEES AFFECTING NURSING PRACTICE

Nurse practice committees, policy/procedure committees (representation from all levels of nursing)

RECOGNITION AND REWARD SYSTEM FOR CLINICAL COMPETENCY

Developed with input from those nurses who will be directly involved

RECOGNITION AND PERSONNEL BENEFITS

Employee retention and reward committee or task force (multidisciplinary approach)

AVAILABILITY OF NURSING LIBRARY

Books, periodicals, and literature search capabilities via computer

SUGGESTION PROGRAM FOR NURSING

Suggestions or recommendations that have been successfully implemented on a nursing unit are shared with other units with credit given to the originator, and assistance is given if further development or patent is indicated

MANAGEMENT TRAINING

Human processes skills, functions, and management team orientation

CERTIFICATION

Recognition of professional achievement in a specific practice arena (financial compensation for certification merit)

JOINT PRACTICE COMMITTEES

---

creased job satisfaction. It is important to note that the *opportunity* (including all types of opportunity) has been shown to be a very important determinant impacting on turnover. In fact, one study has found opportunity to be four times as important as *pay*.[22]

Opportunity for promotion. Opportunities for promotion do not occur frequently in most hospitals. When they do occur, it is imperative that staff be informed of all vacancies and that applications of interested candidates be handled in a fair and equitable manner. The head nurse not only concentrates on factors consistent with his or her professional development but also on the development of an assistant. The role of mentor is rarely seen on the nurse manager's job description, but it is an expectation of every nurse manager that time and attention be devoted to the development of a successor for that position.

Clinical, managerial, educational, and specialist options

Institutions across the country have developed different types of career ladder concepts to attract and retain professional nurses. Some hospitals have been successful with two-track programs (clinical and managerial); others have used three-track or four-track programs with success. The greater successes with career ladder concepts have occurred in institutions where the job descriptions, evaluation tools, and criteria for advancement have been developed by nurse practice committees composed of staff nurse representatives from all areas of nursing. For the purpose of recognizing all possibilities, the four-track career ladder will be discussed here (see Table 5-1).

Clinical ladder concept. There have always been caring, dedicated nurses within the profession who desired to remain in the clinical area at the patient's bedside throughout their entire work life. Financial pressures have often forced them to seek managerial positions in order to upgrade their salary. The traditional and sole recognition in many hospitals has been promotion to a "management position." Few nurses are prepared for management by education, interest, or special training; as a result, many fail in this position. It has only been in the last decade that hospitals have begun to realize that provisions need to be made to retain experienced, competent nurses in the clinical setting and to reward them appropriately. In 1982, the difference in salary between a new graduate and a nurse with 20 years of experience was only about $2000.[8] Such inequities in reward and recognition cannot be allowed to continue.

In the clinical ladder concept, measurable, progressive behaviors that are consistently employed by nurses can be identified, collected, categorized, and used for promotion; the essence of the program is progression through peer review. Quality nursing care can be documented through the initiation of clinical ladders. The concept of clinical ladders envisions and encompasses a system of promotion that can recognize the professional nurse's clinical knowledge, competence, and performance. Advancement in clinical ladders is parallel and complementary to administrative promotion. It offers nurses choices for their career advancement as their interest, motivation, and competence evolve.

TABLE 5-1

Career ladder tracks*

Clinical	Managerial	Educational	Specialist (MSN)
Clinical nurse III ↑	Assistant director of nursing ↑	Director of education ↑	Clinical specialist— coordinator for management
Clinical nurse II ↑	Departmental supervisor ↑	Assistant director of education ↑	Clinical specialist— staff development
Clinical nurse I ↑	Head nurse ↑	Education instructor (MSN) ↑	Clinical specialist— patient education
Clinical nurse (ENTRY)	Assistant head nurse	Education instructor (BSN)	Clinical specialist— unit or department

*It should be noted that whereas the clinical, managerial, and educational tracks are hierarchical, the clinical specialist options all appear on the same organizational level.

The advantage of the clinical ladder system is the provision of a system that rewards practicing (bedside) nurses according to their accomplishments. Indirect benefits to the nurse include improved personal and professional satisfaction, increased motivation, and increased positive attitudes toward self, role, and organization. Advantages to the organization (and nurses themselves) include decreased turnover. In addition, primary nursing interfaces very well with the clinical ladder concept and is the logical and natural extension of such a program. The individual nurse is usually aware of the demands and responsibilities expected when moving from the clinical to the managerial role and has the option to choose whether or not this is a viable career goal for self. This should be a choice based on professional goals and aspirations rather than financial necessity. All nurses are not management material, nor should this be expected. Career ladder strategies recognize personal individuality while providing a mechanism for advancement.

Managerial option. It is incumbent on nursing administration in hospitals to identify nurses who have leadership skills and interests, and to enhance their development through educational programs and provision of preceptors or mentors.

The beginning level of supervision has often been the assistant head nurse. This individual is often in charge of the nursing unit on the evening (3 to 11) or night (11 to 7) shift, or on those days the head nurse is absent. Unfortunately, this nurse usually has no managerial background, limited orientation to the role, and sees the head nurse or supervisor only minimally. This can result in management by hit or miss, insecurity, and often inept leadership. Viable processes for facilitating the growth of these nurses include presupervisory training and assessment, committee assignment, managerial mentors, and supervisory and management training programs. Leadership potential must be identified, rewarded, and refined through staff development.

If nurses in managerial roles in hospitals, or those who aspire to these roles, are expected to succeed, they must be provided with managerial training. This is especially true for those who have not had formal leadership training in their basic nursing programs. Some essential topics are as follows:

Understanding the hospital as a business
Budgets
Staffing
Productivity
Management controls
Interpersonal relations
Human resource management
Communications
Interdependence
Quality assurance
Goal setting
Establishing priorities
Feedback
Performance appraisal
Team building (see Chapter 3)

Educational option. A nurse's inclination toward the educational aspect of nursing can be fulfilled in a variety of settings: hospital, junior college, university, or private consulting business. For the purposes of this discussion only the education track as it pertains to hospitals will be considered. In hospitals today the nursing education department has changed from providing only in-service training to a department that encompasses (1) staff development, (2) orientation, (3) in-service education, (4) continuing education, and (5) community service.

One area often overlooked in staff development programs is that of educational instructor as consultant. Building on skills they already possess, education instructors can make a smooth transition to this role; with appropriate education of the nursing staff to the consultative aspect of their role, they can become valuable resources. As consultants they can appropriately be assigned to the evening and night shifts and will thus be accessible to more nursing personnel.

The primary responsibility for most hospital nursing education departments today is in the area of orientation, that is, assisting the new employee or new graduate nurse in adapting to the institution. However, the focus needs to be redirected toward more emphasis on staff development. Often the department is titled, "Human Resources Development," thus emphasizing its basic purpose. It is important that the education department be included and involved in nursing meetings to facilitate communication, sharing, and data gathering, because this will result in more accepted, relevant, and influential staff development programs.

Clinical specialist/advanced practitioner option. The categories and numbers of nurses with advanced education are increasing and there has been much discussion about the applicability of their skills in the hospital setting. The utilization and cost effectiveness of these persons requires creative thinking on the part of nursing administrators, because until now they have been almost exclusively utilized in primary care settings. Some nursing directors welcome these advanced registered nurse practitioners whereas others consider them impractical.

Some specialist/advanced practitioner categories frequently seen today include the following:

Certified registered nurse anesthetists (CRNA)

Nurse midwives

Pediatric nurse practitioners

Geriatric nurse practitioners

Family planning nurse practitioners

Clinical specialists:

Maternal-child health

Psychiatric

Medical-surgical

Cardiovascular

Emergency/trauma

Because a position of this type is new to the hospital setting, the nursing director, along with the specialist, is responsible for designing a fit within the nursing division. To facilitate maximum utilization of this highly trained nurse, the following components are essential:

1. The specialist develops his or her own job description with input from other members of the nursing staff.
2. Open trust and acceptance of this individual are essential.
3. Creativity on the part of the specialist in relating to nursing staff and hospital administration is recognized.
4. Flexibility in job performance and independence in practice are imperative.
5. Clearly defined areas of responsibility and accountability are outlined.

Personal and interpersonal growth

Personal growth. Personal growth is a concern for nurse leaders as it relates to both themselves and their staff. Growth, development, and change are really only possible from within the individual. The institution and the professional, however, have the responsibility to provide a climate conducive to the personal growth of the practitioner. The responsibility for ongoing professionalization through personal growth is uniquely individual. Much of a nurse's personal growth occurs not in dramatic ways but rather as subtle changes over time brought about by a continuous process of growth, maturity, learning, and change.

For the nurse manager, personal growth is prompted within an organizational milieu where the limits of authority and the areas of responsibility and accountability are defined. Nursing leaders within the organization determine attitudes and behaviors that are appropriate and set the examples that others emulate.

> Five policies (are) essential for such a climate. (1) Subordinates need to know what is expected of them. (2) They need opportunities for development. (3) They need to know how well they are doing. (4) They should be provided with assistance when necessary. (5) They should receive adequate recognition for the results of their efforts.[13]

It is difficult to grow personally or professionally without some picture of oneself. This picture is typically presented by way of feedback gathered from others. Limited as we are by our socialization, we find it difficult and uncomfortable, even improper to present co-workers with feedback, concern, or counsel regarding their personal "selves." Observations regarding personal style, grooming techniques, presentation of self, interpersonal behavior—from positive and negative postures—tend to be left unsaid or gossiped about rather than authentically shared. Personal style impacts on all interactions, including work. It is appropriate that goals for personal growth (and change) be explored and facilitated as a part of the work relationship.

Collegiality among nurses. Nurses have little problem in caring for *clients* in our health care institutions, but when it comes to caring for their *colleagues* as co-workers and fellow nurses, there have been problems. Nurses in general tend to display nonsupportive behavior toward other nurses. This is especially true for those colleagues who have different ideas about patient care or who have difficulty coping with the stress and demands of today's hospitals. This lack of support or helping relationship permeates all of nursing, from nurse administrator to staff nurse. The reasons for this and the "cure" still elude nurses at all levels. Theories abound: (1) lack of confidence among nurses as professional caregivers to colleagues, (2) role ambiguity, (3) lack of public value and trust, (4) lack of interpersonal skills, (5) lack of investment, (6) lack of any such expectation. (See discussion of helping relationships in Chapter 3.) Collegiality connotes sharing, investing, equality, commonality, and in some fashion, stability. Authentic, confronting peer relationships take time to develop. It is difficult to decide which statement is accurate: high turnover reduces collegiality or low collegial relations increase turnover. One definitely compounds the other. As professionals, nurses are responsible to the public for services rendered by all members of the profession. They have a responsibility to practice in accordance with certain standards and codes of ethics. One of the best ways to promote excellence in practice is to provide peer support, guidance, direction, and criticism. This is a cornerstone for professionalism.

Ethics, morals, values. Every nursing relationship begins with an unusual burden of ethical responsibility. Whereas patients may have chosen their physician, they do not usually have the option of choosing their nurse. The dependency of patienthood has to be based on the assumption that care will be offered that is, at the very least, safe, effective, and morally responsible. Frequently morals and ethics are equated, yet there are important differences. *Morality* is generally thought of as behavior according to custom or tradition. *Ethics*, by contrast, is the free rational assessment of courses of action in relation to principles and rules of conduct. Hence most nursing practice decisions are ethical ones. Ethical practices that underlie the foundation of nursing professional relationships originate from several sources. Among these are human rights, commitment to the public welfare, nursing peer professional affiliations, and a commitment to nurse-client relationships.

A *value* is a personal belief or attitude about the truth, beauty, or worth of any thought, object, or behavior. A belief is not a value unless it is freely chosen. Values play major parts in how a supervisory nurse deals with subordinates; unless a supervisor understands and appreciates the values of employees, effective supervision will not be possible. How one performs as a nurse depends on one's values. Personal values and ethics, as well as professional morals, combine to form one's philosophy of nursing. Every nurse needs to develop a philosophy of nursing as a part of his or her personal and interpersonal growth. Too often nursing decisions need to be made that should be drawn from a philosophy of nursing when none has been formulated. Today, a nurse's philosophy of nursing has to grapple with many controversial issues, including euthanasia, abortion, death with dignity, and professional incompetence.

Passages. Only in the last 5 to 10 years has very much attention been given the developmental periods in early and middle adulthood and addressed in such books as Levinson's *The Seasons of a Man's Life* and Sheehy's *Passages*. These developmental stages have implications for both the nurse practitioner and the nurse manager. A knowledge of these predictable periods in adult life with respect to nurses will help practitioners and managers cope with midlife crisis through such activities as career planning and change, support groups, and self-understanding.

A list of questions that facilitate "reappraising the past" and that can be addressed by individuals as a part of personal and professional growth during the midlife stage have been adapted from *The Seasons of a Man's Life,* by Daniel J. Levinson. They are listed here:

1. What have I done with my life?
2. What do I really get from and give to my spouse, children, work, friends, and myself?
3. What is it that I truly want for myself and others?
4. What are my central values and how are they being reflected in my life?
5. What are my greatest talents and how am I wasting them or using them?
6. What have I done with my early dream and what do I want to do with it now?
7. Can I live in a way that combines my current desires, values, and talents?
8. How satisfactory is my present life structure, how suitable for the self, how viable in the world, and how shall I change it to provide a basis for the future?

It is not difficult to relate developmental periods to some of the frustrations and disillusionment that nurses experience in early adulthood and midlife transition. The delicate balancing of multiple roles in society and the need for professional recognition and fulfillment often create crises for nurses in their quest for personal and interpersonal growth.

Leadership training

Whose responsibility? Whose responsibility is nurse leadership training? The educational institution? The employing agency? Traditionally, we think of nurses in managerial roles as leaders in hospitals: the assistant head nurse, head nurse, supervisor, and assistant director of nursing. This is a very narrow interpretation of the leader concept, for truly all professional nurses are leaders in the hospital setting. Staff nurses lead nursing assistants, orderlies, licensed practical nurses, student nurses, and many other ancillary employees who provide services to and for patients. Where should the responsibility fall? Diploma and associate degree programs have minimal leadership training and BSN graduates report only a one-semester course on leadership. With so little preparation in such a skill-demanding role, can nurses be expected to exercise leadership in the hospital setting? The direction is clear: hospitals will have to assume the responsibility of providing leadership training. How this is done is a reflection of the value that hospital and nursing administrators place on nurse leaders and the investment they are willing to make in nursing performance and potential. It is extremely relevant that hospitals believe that the return on this investment is *staff nurse retention.*

Basic supervision programs. Hospitals must individualize leadership-supervisory programs and courses to meet the changing needs of the institution. The length of time may vary, but most introductory or basic courses in leadership training require a minimum of 20 hours, which could be divided into 2-hour segments over a 10-week period. Timely topics to be included in this Phase 1 are as follows:

    I. Introduction to supervision
   II. Management by objectives; goal setting
  III. Organizing and staffing
  IV. Communication and the supervisor
   V. Employee needs and motivation
  VI. Performance appraisal: coaching
 VII. Problem solving and the supervisor
VIII. Budgeting
  IX. Daily supervisory activities
   X. Self-development for the supervisor

In order to effect any long-range benefits from leadership training at the beginning of the programs, all first-line supervisors including assistant head nurses, head nurses, and supervisors should receive the same information and must have the opportunity to conduct dialogue around these issues.

Advanced management programs. Following the Phase 1 basic supervisory training for assistant head nurses, head nurses, and supervisors, courses in advanced management skills should be provided to complement and enhance skills introduced in the basic course. The advanced management skills program, primarily geared for head nurses and supervisors, should encompass but not be limited to the following areas.

  I. *Management—a historical perspective*

    Purpose: In exploring the principles of scientific management and the development of management styles, it should be emphasized that bureaucratic management principles have a negative impact on job satisfaction and contribute to rising costs for hospital care. Studies have indicated that a more humanistic and participative approach to patient care by hospital and nursing administration is needed if hospital nursing and hospitals are to survive and provide the intended services. By studying the development of management thought, the nursing manager can define his or her role, develop a philosophy of management, learn tools and techniques for implementing management responsibilities, and gain an increased understanding of how to work with others to accomplish goals.

II. *Interpersonal relations—communications*

Purpose: The reasons the nurse manager must be able to communicate effectively and to develop skills in verbal and nonverbal communication and the art of active listening should be identified. Practice will solidify skills. Communication excellence that enables the nurse leader to represent nursing appropriately in multidisciplinary settings is promoted, and thus encourages development of self-assurance and self-awareness as an interacting member of the health care team.

III. *Leadership—motivation and change*

Purpose: The nurse manager must be provided with the knowledge, skills, and behaviors to put to effective use every available management strategy. Also, as a change agent of the institution, the nurse manager must be introduced to the theories, ethics, and skills of organization development, change agentry, and assessment. The implications of accountability for nursing care, personnel, and fiscal aspects are also significant learning acquisitions.

IV. *Coaching for improved performance*

Purpose: The nurse manager develops skills that can be used to improve employees' performance and behavior through coaching techniques, thus increasing efficiency, productivity, and job satisfaction. Those aspects of performance that are critical to quality of care are identified, and promotive (rather than undermining and reactive) coaching patterns are established.

V. *Employee life cycle concepts*

A. *Interviewing*

Purpose: The nurse manager is allowed to gain skills and insight in personnel selection, both new hires and transfer applicants, for his or her unit. This screening process can reduce turnover, orientation costs, and ultimately, costs per patient day. Opportunities are provided to identify desired personnel attributes and to practice asking questions.

B. *Performance appraisal and counseling*

Purpose: The supervisor learns to assess and critically appraise the employees' work performance. Experience in the utilization of feedback tools is provided via verbal and written communication. Skills are developed that will enhance the growth and development of employees through helping behaviors.

C. *Progressive discipline*

Purpose: The nurse manager is provided a framework to use in selecting options and alternatives for discipline based on employee values and appropriateness of action. Discipline is examined as a positive influence, a useful management problem-solving tool. Consistency, honesty, confidentiality, and immediacy are discussed as key elements in successful discipline.

VI. *Team-building techniques*

Purpose: The nurse manager's knowledge and skills in team-building techniques are increased in order to develop employee and department cohesiveness and effectiveness and to promote job satisfaction through professional collegiality, positive interdependence, and joint problem solving.

VII. *Decision making*

Purpose: The nurse manager is provided the opportunity to study the decision-making process and to practice skills in simulated situations. Decision making in relation to leadership, management, and quality is a primary area of focus.

VIII. *Priority setting*

Purpose: Nurse managers develop concepts of time management and identify their personal and professional values and priorities in order to obtain maximum benefit from time available on the job. They explore time-saving and time-wasting practices. They compare and combine efficiency and effectiveness.

These topics are just a few of the contemporary subjects that can be used as 2-day workshops. Choices depend on individual hospitals' goals and objectives in nurse leadership training. Other pertinent subjects for middle and upper management positions in nursing are staffing; operational, demand, and expense budgets; computer applications in nursing; quality assurance; and risk management.

Selecting appropriate people to promote to the managerial ranks is a concern of executives in all organizations. This concern is no less important in health care institutions, especially among the ranks of executive nursing management. It is important to note that being a nurse manager does not mean that a nurse has given up nursing and will no longer use the skills and knowledge that have been acquired for patient care. Rather, it means that these basic knowledge areas and skills are used in different ways. Demonstrated technical or clinical ability does not ensure effective managerial performance; however, it is an asset to be able to provide technical consultation. Likewise, leadership training does not guarantee leader excellence; but it does improve the odds.

Management potential assessment. The climate characteristics of a nursing department—cooperation, employee satisfaction, turnover, conflict—are greatly influenced by its leadership. A frustrated and ineffective manager has a negative impact on the whole organization. Because choosing the right leader is so important to success, it should be a thoughtful, deliberate process.

To eliminate superficial selection, some hospitals have followed industry's example and identified and developed managers through an ongoing process. This concept, the management potential assessment, is a systematic method of identifying and targeting head nurses–patient care coordinators–managers of tomorrow. This capability of identifying high-potential *promotable* persons provides supervisory talent for succession work force planning to meet the long-range plans of nursing administration (see Chapter 2 on career plan). It is also a way to avoid turnover resulting from frustrated career ambitions. The program, which can be tailored to the institution's needs, can be simple or sophisticated depending on the setting and financial resources of the institution. Assessors can be selected from available resources within nursing administration. The program is developed by defining qualities to be measured and developing the tools to be employed.

The assessment center concept ideally takes potential candidates for promotion away from the work place and exposes them to simulated experiences that illustrate situations encountered in specific managerial roles. Simulation exercises include decision making and problem solving, conflict resolution, counseling, coaching, and other areas pertinent to the managerial position being assessed. Standardized exercises are usually administered by assessors who are several management levels above those being assessed. This provides opportunities for evaluations of candidates under controlled (laboratory) conditions and makes comparative judgments possible.

The number of candidates for this program will vary with the institution but usually ranges from 6 to 12 with an assessor/candidate ratio of from 1:1 to 1:3. Length of the program will vary usually from 1 to 3 full days. A program designed to help select a nurse for a management position will be shorter than one designed to develop strengths and identify weaknesses. This type of program has been most successful with identification of potential head nurse candidates. It must be flexible and comprehensive in covering desired managerial characteristics. It must also attend to issues of confidentiality and individual differences within the organization.

Exercises used in assessment programs may include but are by no means limited to the following:

1. Personal interview
2. In-basket exercise
3. Leaderless group discussions
4. Problem analysis
5. Issues discussion (e.g., appropriate discipline)
6. Mock selection interview
7. Ethical dilemmas in supervision

Participants for assessment programs are most often nominated by their supervisors based on their past performance and potential for advancement, although some organizations allow employees at a certain level, meeting certain criteria, to nominate themselves. The objectives of nurse management potential assessment centers have been stated by Mark Silber Associates, Ltd., hospital management psychologists:[25]

- To identify and target staff nurses with managerial promotion potential
- To guide Nursing Administration in manpower succession planning for the Nursing Division futurism
- To provide a vehicle of career guidance for these high potential persons . . . the goal is retention
- To provide a dual focus: Increasing present effectiveness and preparing persons for tomorrow's manager requirements
- To implement a systematic program that utilizes objective data collection processes
- To improve the cost-effectiveness of nurse manager identification
- Prediction: Which nurses to count on for managing tomorrow?

The qualities to be measured in such a program can be selected from the American Management Association's multimedia supervisory course and modified to meet those required in the head nurse role. Although the management potential assessment is certainly not a panacea for the nurse management selection process, it is a method that can be a welcome adjunct when used in combination with other selection tools. Although new and additional burdens of accountability have been placed on the nurse manager, preparation for the new role has not kept pace. It behooves nurse managers at all levels to reassess and upgrade their knowledge, skills, and performance to meet the changing expectations and to be accountable for providing excellent health care.

There are no formulas that can give a nursing director the answer to how much leadership training is relevant, meaningful, or even necessary for the staff. It is a personal and institutional investment, and thus an individual agency decision. Achieving desirable outcomes in the areas of patient care and of personnel and fiscal management is the result of effective nursing management.

INDIVIDUALITY AND JOB DESIGN CONSIDERATIONS

Nurses frequently report ambivalent feelings about nursing—a love/hate relationship that sometimes spans an entire career. They love working with patients but they hate working conditions in hospitals. Providing good nursing care is far more difficult than it should be because of poor communication, lack of appreciation, and conflicts with physicians and management.

One of the most important tasks facing hospital leadership is to create, develop, and maintain a working climate that stimulates rather than stifles employees. Hospitals in the past have not assigned the same priority and prominence to staff development as they have to productivity, finance, and marketing. One of the main reasons employees, especially qualified ones, leave a company is because management fails to understand or chooses not to pay attention to their basic needs. There appears to be a large gap between what hospital management thinks employees want and what they actually desire.

It is the responsibility of the director of nursing service and the supervisory personnel to creatively design or redesign the work of nursing to make and keep hospitals attractive to nurses. In order to provide programs and opportunities for nurses that meet their needs, their needs must first be ascertained. This can be done through an attitude survey of nurses within the agency and also of nurses who are licensed actively or inactively within the community. (Such a list can be obtained from state boards of nursing.)

Flexible scheduling

Unique ways have been developed by hospitals to encourage professional nurses with personal or family commitments that limit their availability to work traditional schedules to return to the hospital. Such programs include the following.

Shared jobs. Two part-time nurses fill one full-time position.

Half-shifts. Two nurses fill an 8-hour shift, each working 4 hours.

Float and PRN pools within hospital. Allow nurses to choose the days and shifts they are able to work; it is less restrictive than regular part-time employment. This concept was patterned after the supplemental staffing agencies that meet nurses' needs for flextime, but often compound staffing problems for hospitals.

Flextime. The concept of flextime has numerous variations, including the following:

1. Eight-hour shifts at nontraditional times (e.g., 9 AM to 5 PM; 10 AM to 6 PM; 11 AM to 7 PM)
2. Less than an 8-hour shift at staggered hours usually during busiest time of day
3. Baylor modification of flextime (see below)
4. Seven days on/seven days off
5. Four 10-hour shifts per week

Flextime may be defined as a form of alternate staffing that seeks to meet the needs of the individual while at the same time satisfying the requirements of the organization. The concept has been used extensively in Japan and Europe and since 1973 has been used in the United States by a number of industries. More recently an adaptation of flextime has been used by Baylor University Medical Center in Dallas and is being copied by other health care institutions across the country. The Baylor modification of flextime involves the utilization of special nursing personnel who work two 12-hour shifts on Saturdays and Sundays and receive the pay and compensation of having worked a 40-hour work week. Other staff then work a Monday-through-Friday, 5-day/40-hour week.

Some of the results reported by hospitals who have used flexible scheduling are as follows:

1. Agency nurse utilization has been either decreased or eliminated altogether.
2. Success in recruitment has increased, markedly decreasing staff vacancies.
3. Costs for flexible scheduling have been offset by the reduced use of outside agency staff.
4. Nursing staff satisfaction with scheduling is high, thereby increasing the stability of staff.

The cost figure for a hospital with flexible scheduling increased overall salary expense by about 2%.[7]

Flextime, shared jobs, or PRN (as needed) staffing is impossible without flexibility and creative thinking in staffing and scheduling. The skills and knowledge of nonemployed nurses are needed by hospitals; this flexibility allows these nurses to reenter the work force and practice their profession, but does not put unreasonable strain on external relationships and responsibilities.

Job redesign and job enrichment

The first serious modern management thinker to redesign jobs was Frederick Taylor. He discovered while studying jobs in the early 1900s that a worker's output would increase if planning and controlling aspects of the job were removed, leaving the person to perform the job. Thus a new wave of job specialization began, emphasizing efficiency through repetitiveness and standardization. The movement also brought into the job setting boredom, monotony, increased absenteeism, and turnover. This has led to the contemporary movement to redesign or enrich jobs in an effort to improve morale, productivity, and retention. The concept has found favorable application in labor-intensive industries and has recently generated interest in the possibility of applying it to nurse retention.

Frederick Herzberg, although not without critics, conducted in-depth research in the mid 1950s that has application for nursing. Herzberg stated that there were two sets of conditions necessary to satisfy employees. The first set, the hygiene factors, includes such aspects as good working conditions, job security, realistic company policies, adequate salaries, and good supervision —all of which tend to comprise a healthy work environment conducive to job satisfaction. The second set, motivational factors, include recognition, responsibility, advancement, and salary increases. These motivational factors will not in themselves bring job satisfaction, but when coupled with hygiene factors bring rewards in terms of employee retention, increased productivity, improved morale, and the creation of a positive work climate. Examples of motivators and hygiene factors are listed below.

Motivators	Hygiene factors
Achievement	Company policy
Work itself	Supervision
Responsibility	Working conditions
Recognition	Salary
Advancement	Job security
Growth	Status
Control of work	Personal life

The application of the motivation-hygiene theory is referred to most often as job enrichment. Attention to the role of hygiene factors, as begun by Herzberg, has played a key role in current job redesign programs. Factors that must be understood by managers in altering jobs were proposed by Oldham, Hackman, and Pearce[19a]:

1. When employees are well satisfied with the hygiene factors and have strong needs for personal growth through the job, job redesign has very favorable effects on work satisfaction, performance, and motivation.
2. When employees are well satisfied with the hygiene factors but have weak needs for personal growth through work, job enrichment has only moderate effects on satisfaction, performance, and motivation.
3. When employees are dissatisfied with the hygiene factors and have weak needs for personal growth through work, job enrichment has no effect on satisfaction, performance, and motivation.

The term job enrichment has also been used as a version of the Japanese industrial model, which encourages employees to be generalists as opposed to specialists, mastering a number of jobs within the organization. As applied to health care, nurses have been encouraged to request transfers to other nursing units or departments within the hospital, allowing them to learn new skills, to be associated with different physicians and nurse colleagues, and to broaden their perspectives about the organization. Job enrichment has been a factor in countering the burnout syndrome.

Quality circles are just beginning to be implemented in American health care institutions. This technique, originated by the Japanese, represents an attempt to elicit employee involvement in problem solving and quality assurance. It is too early to claim successes from this technique, but it appears to have merit in that it provides a mechanism for employee involvement in the assessment of quality of care, the appropriateness of care, and peer review.

PERCEIVED JOB REDESIGN BENEFITS

Feeling that nurses are a part of the patient care team
Working the shift of choice
Assignments consistent with training and experience
Availability of nurse preceptors at the clinical unit level
Knowing work schedules a month in advance through cyclical scheduling
Flexible scheduling, flextime
Participatory management programs that give nurses a say in nursing administration
Joint nurse-physician committees to discuss patient care
Availability of education instructors to be used for consultation

---

The key to sustained motivation seems to lie in assignments that push people to the limits of their abilities and that provide them with new and serious challenges. Dissatisfaction is part of humanness because today's motivations will be tomorrow's expectations. Nurses are not objects on a staffing board but are valuable assets whose individual needs and requirements must be assessed and then blended with the needs of the hospital and the patient (see above).

PROGRAM DESIGN

A chapter focusing on ongoing professionalization implies some type of continuous movement toward becoming a professional. To a great extent, this movement depends on something happening inside an organization. It is true that some activities occurring outside the formal organization impact on professionalism, and these have been explored throughout this chapter. It is believed that what goes on *inside* an organization or institution will have more of an impact on turnover and retention. Training and growth going on inside a group will have the effect of further melding that group and increasing the individual's feelings of cohesiveness and belongingness. This effect does not come about by accident, however.

> Whether one is planning a course in human relations, a weekend personal growth laboratory, or a management development seminar, there are common concerns and questions that need to be considered in order for an optimum design to emerge.[21]

In order to plan and carry out a program of ongoing training within a hospital, two important questions must be answered:
- What will be the content?
- What will be the process?

Certain skills are necessary for success in carrying out training programs, and these must be present to some extent in the training staff, whether the staff is in-house or augmented by professionals from the outside. "It is helpful to break your potential staff into two groups: those with special content expertise and those with skills for assisting the learning process."[5] Of the two, content expertise is probably easier to obtain. A person competent in *process* complements the content expert by helping to design a program that will solidify the knowledge imparted. As will be discussed later, central to any program content is a statement of objectives. The objective(s) should be more specifically stated than "to help in team building" or "for organizational development."

There are no specific recommendations here for the *content* to be covered in the training programs; the possibilities are nearly infinite. Specific content must be dictated by the needs of the organizations.

The beauty of a well-designed program (*process*) is that it gets results regardless of the *content*. The content is important, certainly, but well-designed and well-selected training exercises will have a number of spinoff results in the form of better understanding of the organization, greater sense of personal worth, and enhanced individual motivation.

When speaking here of ongoing professionalism, we should perhaps admonish the reader. Throughout the book, we have either indicated or implied that there are forces seesawing nurses in sometimes opposing directions; that job conditions do not fall neatly into one management/motivational theory or the other. For instance, in Chapter 4, it is noted that nurses are working on the upper levels of Maslow's hierarchy of needs without having fulfilled the lower level needs. The same type of apparent anomaly may be encountered in dealing with the problems of nursing professionalism and turnover. Several research studies quoted and/or discussed by Price and Mueller[23] suggest that increased professionalism *may* result in greater turnover. Although empirical results are not too strong and application of the research to nursing is even more scanty, there is at least a possibility that it may be true. One interpretation of the results is that as a group becomes more professional, the individual's loyalties are linked more with the profession than with the employing institution. Within the nursing profession there already appears to be precious little loyalty to the institution and little more to the profession. Suppose that the hypothesis relating turnover to professionalism is true. Two thoughts immediately come to mind:

1. Turnover at unacceptable rates already exists. Professionalism is not the major force in turnover except in an ancillary manner. If the suggestions in this book are carried out, they can have a dramatic effect in decreasing turnover. It is believed that an offsetting increase in turnover due to increasing professionalism would be a small increment compared to this decrease.

2. If turnover exists, which is best for the hospital: to contend with the turnover of personnel who are not very professional, or to know that newly hired personnel will be from a pool that is continually more and more professional? It is therefore more likely that institutions supporting the professional development of nurses will enhance their reputation among nurses at the very least and may increase nurses' loyalty and commitment to staying.

The mere expenditure of funds to bring in or conduct training programs will not suffice. The engagement of a big name in the field (any field) without regard to the applicability of the program's content to the specific organization and the people therein may do more harm than good. The members of the organization may see this as a wasting of funds that could better be utilized in salary enhancement. "We emphasize that it is the individual's values, expectations, and *perception of internal development opportunities* that guide their turnover decision"[19] (italics added). Generalized training or specific training that is inappropriate to the group will not be seen in a good light.

The types of designs used for training programs will depend a great deal on (1) the type of organization now in place, (2) the present development of the organization, and (3) the stage of development of each person within the organization. The final criterion for assessing any proposed training program stated is: Does the training impact positively on and congruently with the organization, its goals, and its human resources? This question is valid whether the training is carried out internally or externally, by inside or outside consultants or trainers.

Training is accomplished by many different methods. The method selected must be tailored not only to the general audience (e.g., nurses, physicians, managers), but also to the type of content to be imparted and to the specific individuals in the group to be trained. Few generalities are possible. Some people learn best from written material, some from oral presentation and explanation, and others from hands-on demonstration. In general, however, most people learn best when learning by doing, that is, when they are given a chance to practice in some manner what they are supposed to learn. (See the discussion in Chapter 8 on experiential learning for more specific input regarding this learning theory.) This rule, like all others, has exceptions. In general, the best program design will not limit itself to any one method but will tailor the method to people and situations.

The gamut of possible methods extends from little participation to full participation by the individuals involved; from presentations (lectures) to participant determination and conducting of the agenda. Though each has its own advantages and disadvantages, the important concept is that each will work if based on the goals and needs of the group.

No longer can the requirements for training claim to be satisfied by (almost) random selection of a program because its title or outline "sounds good." In order to carry out true training, a multistep approach must be employed in a *continuous feedback loop*. Any well-designed program of training follows a logical series of steps; however, it must be recognized that after the initial start-up, several of the steps may be going on at any one time in different components of the program. Roughly, the steps and their order are as follows:

1. *Recognition of the need.* Before any program can be initiated, there must be a felt need somewhere in the organization. The need may be stated or sensed but someone must be aware there is a need for something to be done. In the case of nursing turnover, the need has already been felt and expressed. The turnover rate is unacceptable; monetary and other costs are too high to continue.

2. *Data gathering and assessment.* Some indication must be available of where in the organization the needs are, their extent, and the stage of development of the group for which a need has been identified. Data may be taken from several different sources:
   • Individual consultations and informal chats with group members
   • Group sessions where members are encouraged to air their concerns regarding the organization. The success of such sessions presupposes that members are comfortable enough *with* the group and *as* a group to express opinions.
   • More formal or structured interviews
   • Questionnaires that assess the atmosphere and conditions of the group and organization

3. *Program design.* Once the above information is available, the actual design can begin. Training devices selected will depend greatly on the needs to be filled. Some needs strictly for knowledge, for instance, may be filled most quickly by the traditional lecture approach. In general, however, except for limited applications, it is recommended that experiential learning exercises be emphasized. (Again, see Chapter 8 for further discussions regarding experiential learning.) Several excellent manuals or series of manuals are available (see the Pfeiffer and Jones *Annual Handbooks for Group Facilitators*,[21] for instance), giving various exercises of differing complexity and objectives. The general purposes of exercises are usually stated. Some activities may be adapted to *other training uses*, but in general this should be attempted by a fairly confident and competent trainer. Each activity to be used should be selected based on several criteria:
   • Is it appropriate to the need discerned in the data-gathering phase above?
   • Is it appropriate to the group? Are group members comfortable enough

with themselves and each other to carry out the activity, benefit from it, and understand the results?

- Is it appropriate to the background and expertise of the trainer? Some activities should be carried out only by a very experienced trainer who can ascertain and facilitate functional group action.
- Is it appropriate at this point in the training process, considering the training activities that have been previously accomplished and those that are to follow?

When the activities have been selected, they can be woven into a coherent training pattern. At this step, it must be recognized that "in general, training activities need to follow each other in psychological, learner-centered sequence, rather than in a purely logical progression."[18] Training activities must be put into a sequence that allows members of the group to grow and progress both individually and as a group, at a speed acceptable to them.

4. *Reassessment.* At *regular* points in the training, recycling is necessary and assessment is essential. For instance, if one or two new members enter the group, activities may be necessary to allow them to become acclimated and to join the group before further training is attempted. At discrete times in the training, the facilitator must stop and conduct an assessment of the group and where it is in development. Such an assessment is critical in determining where to go next.

The trainer must be experienced enough to recognize when there is a need to change directions, and to do so as needed. There should be no reluctance to follow an unplanned tangent if the need arises. The trainer must be strong enough and skilled in knowing when to begin "leaving the groups," allowing the group an increasingly greater hand in designing and accomplishing its own training activities.

In order to be more certain that the training used in the organization is (1) applicable to the individuals for whom it is intended, (2) needed for developmental purposes, and (3) appropriate to the long-term goals of the organization, it is wise to hire someone as director of training. Such a person must have professional training as a facilitator and be cognizant of program designing, assessment tools, training methods, and expertise available both inside and outside the organization. This person must be responsible for knowing the organization-specific needs to which training is to be applied. By coordinating all training, the director assures that the organization's money will be well spent.

A CONCEPTUAL CONCLUSION

The responsibility for ongoing professionalism is something that each practitioner of the profession must accept individually as a personal commitment. However, that responsibility in a unique way rests on nurse managers. Only when the demand for excellence in the profession is unequivocally stated, conscientiously maintained, and suitably rewarded, will hospitals and nursing be able to attract and keep practitioners who are qualified and committed assets to the profession.

REFERENCES AND ADDITIONAL READINGS

1. Blake, R.R., and Mouton, J.S.: The new managerial Grid, Houston, 1979, Gulf Publishing Co.
2. Calkin, J.D.: Let's rethink staff development programs, J. Nurs. Admin. **9**(2):16-19, June 1979.
3. Clifford, J.C.: Managerial control versus professional autonomy: a paradox, J. Nurs. Admin. **11**(9):19-21, Sept. 1981.
4. Curtin, L., and Flaherty, M.J.: Nursing ethics theories and pragmatics, Bowie, Md., 1982, Robert J. Brady Co.
5. Davis, L.N.: Planning, conducting, and evaluating workshops, Austin, Texas, 1974, Learning Concepts.
6. Devereaux, P.M.: Nurse/physician collaboration: nursing practice considerations, J. Nurs. Admin. **11**(9):37-39, Sept. 1981.
7. Dison, C.C., Carter, N., and Bromley, P.: Making the change to flextime, Am. J. Nurs. **81**(12):2162-2164, Dec. 1981.
8. Donovan, L.: Survey of nursing incomes: part two. What increases income most, RN **43**:27-30, Feb. 1980.
9. Gerschefski, L.: Assessment and development for head nurse positions, Superv. Nurse **11**(2):21-25, Feb. 1980.
10. Godfrey, M.A., and Nursing '78: Job satisfaction—or should that be dissatisfaction? How nurses feel about nursing. Part one, Nursing '78 Career Guide, April, pp. 90-102.
11. Hatfield, B.: How to develop a complete nursing management program, Hosp. Topics **59**:12-14, March/April 1981.
12. Hill, B.S.: Retention crisis, Nurs. Mgmt. **13**(1):20-21, Jan. 1982.
13. Holle, M.L.: Staff nurse yesterday; nurse manager today, Superv. Nurse **11**(4): 52-56, April 1980.
14. Kernaghan, S.G.: The nurse shortage: how can we turn the exodus around? Hospitals **56**(3):53-56, Feb. 1, 1982.
15. Lysaught, J.P.: Action in affirmation: toward an unambiguous profession of nursing, New York, 1981, McGraw-Hill Book Co.
16. Lysaught, J.P.: Nursing in a changing society, keynote address to opening session, Florida Nurses' Association, Jacksonville, Sept. 11, 1981.
17. Milbourn, G.: A primer on implementing job redesign, Super. Mgmt. **26**(1):27-37, Jan. 1981.
18. Miles, M.B.: Learning to work in groups, New York, 1959, Teachers College Press.
19. Mobley, W.H.: Employee turnover: causes, consequences, and control, Reading, Mass., 1982, Addison-Wesley Publishing Co.
19a. Oldham, G.R., Hackman, J.R., and Pearce, J.L.: Conditions under which employees respond positively to enriched work, J. Appl. Psychol. **61**:397, Aug. 1976.
20. Pannell, M.: Teaching hospitals build models for nursing organizations, Hospitals **56**(3):60-63, Feb. 1, 1982.

21. Pfeiffer, J.W., and Jones, H.E.: Design considerations in laboratory education. In Pfeiffer, J. Williams, and Jones, Hohn E., editors: Annual Handbook for Group Facilitators, La Jolla, Calif., 1973.

22. Price, J.L., and Mueller, C.W.: A causal model of turnover for nurses, Acad. Mgmt. J. **24**(3):543-565, 1981.

23. Price, J.L., and Mueller, C.W.: Professional turnover: the case of nurses, Jamaica, N.Y., 1981, Spectrum Publications.

24. Sigmon, P.M.: Clinical ladders and primary nursing: the wedding of the two, Nurs. Admin. Quart. **3**(3):63-67, Spring 1981.

25. Silber, M.: Promotional brochure, 1981, Mark Silber Associates, Ltd.

26. Sleicher, M.: Nursing is not a profession, Nurs. Health Care **2**:186-191, April 1981.

27. Traska, M.R.: Nurses as managers: acceptance problems may lie with nurses themselves, Hospitals **56**(3):57-59, Feb. 1, 1982.

28. Ulsasar-Van Lanen, J.: Lateral promotion keeps skilled nurses in direct patient care, Hospitals **55**(5):87-90, March 1, 1981.

29. Weisman, C.S., Alexander, C.S., and Morlock, L.L.: Hospital decision making: what is nursing's role? J. Nurs. Admin. **11**(9):31-35, Sept. 1981.

6

THE HOSPITAL MILIEU

The hospital milieu is confusing, complex, and emotionally charged. Contributing to the complicated environment is the triumvirate made up of hospital board, medical staff, and hospital administration who seek to comanage the institution. The degree of cooperation and the assignment of authority and power to each of the three groups varies considerably from institution to institution, depending on the relative involvement of the three governing groups, the type of hospital operation, and the financial condition. Each of these variables constrains or enhances the involvement of the three groups.

A major reassessment and redefinition of the roles and responsibilities of each member of this triad occurred in the 1960s. During this time, the pressures for more egalitarian, humanistic, and shared organizational management became felt. Additionally, with the increased visibility of women, nursing began to have significant impact on the hospital's administration. At the same time, the *Darling* decision (*Darling* vs. *Charleston Community Memorial Hospital*) in 1965 began to define legally the liability of a hospital for the quality of care it renders. This and other more recent court cases have increased pressure on the governing bodies of hospitals for responsible leadership and control. Decisions against the hospital have resulted in settlements of six to seven figures, inflating already alarming malpractice insurance premiums. Adverse publicity has placed hospitals at a disadvantage in protecting their image and finances. Consequently, the triumvirate has been changing.

Alterations in the composition and relationships among the governing bodies of health care institutions have caused changes and pressures throughout the institution. Changes in the external environment (consumer, political, legal) have put the caregivers, from executive level to staff nurse, in responding postures. Consequences are felt in the organization in terms of relations within and among departments, in terms of accountability in the organization, and in terms of the structure of the organization itself. This chapter explores these issues and others affecting the hospital's milieu.

At a cursory level, the three governing groups are related in the traditional hierarchical arrangement (Fig. 6-1). The typical governance structure of a voluntary, not-for-profit hospital is as follows:
- Board of trustees/directors (and committees) who make overall policy decisions
- Medical staff committees and chiefs of service (surgical, medical, obstetrical, etc.) who recommend and implement policy concerning medical services
- Hospital administrators who recommend and implement policy concerning support and financial services and who define relationships between medical and support services and the hospital

The governing bodies in a for-profit hospital are roughly the same. In a

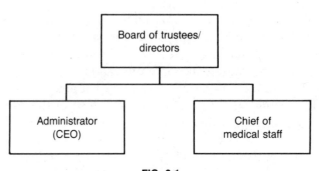

FIG. 6-1
Typical governance structure of a voluntary, not-for-profit hospital.

multihospital corporation, however, the above structure at the hospital level is overlaid with a superstructure at the corporate level. The day-to-day operations and relations are similar in either case. Thus the discussion to follow is applicable to most hospital circumstances.

In order to understand the role and responsibility of these groups more fully and to put the hospital milieu in proper perspective as it relates to nurse retention, each of these three governing groups is examined separately.

ADMINISTRATION: BOARD OF TRUSTEES/DIRECTORS

The board of trustees/directors is the policy-making body of a hospital. Members may be active, using their knowledge and expertise to be involved in hospital affairs, or they may be passive by abdicating their responsibility to the administrative staff (i.e., the administrator, assistants, and department heads).

The hospital industry in the United States is facing a series of challenges, with serious problems arising from within the hospital (medical staff accountability, nursing shortages), within the industry (competition, overbedding, new technology), and from the outside (government, consumer awareness, legal implications). These areas include but a few of the many issues that will have to be addressed by hospital governing boards. How a board chooses to approach these issues and the manner in which the issues are handled have a direct bearing on the future performance of governing boards and of the hospitals for which they are responsible.

The reaction of a board to any of these issues is highly dependent on its membership. The composition of a hospital's governing board may take many forms. A traditional approach is to have the board composed of prominent members of the community, people who have attained high status in business or the professions. Also members of families of "old wealth" are often found on hospital boards. More recently there has been a move to appoint individuals as trustees for their expertise or for their leadership ability. This is seen when a public relations expert or a powerful community leader is chosen who can wield power and sway public opinion for the hospital cause. Some hospitals, in an attempt to promote the spirit of "consumerism," have appointed health care consumers who have none of the previously mentioned qualifications, but who do have a sincere desire to serve their community.

The relationship of the board of trustees of a hospital to the administration of the institution cannot be fully understood without first having an understanding of the nature of its role. There must be an awareness on the part of those who appoint or elect hospital trustees of the significance of the appointment. A board holds a hospital in trust. In order to fulfill this trust, it is the ultimate source of authority. By exercising this authority, the appointed individual, through his or her contribution or impediment to pertinent health care issues, can positively or negatively influence the future course of the health care institution and of the community and consumers it serves. Thus the composition of a hospital board can make the difference between a backward hospital that stagnates and handicaps the community it serves, and a progressive one that meets contemporary health challenges head-on.

Hospital trustees should be citizens who can willingly and freely devote their time and energy to the cause of improving the quality of health care for the members of their community. In the past, appointment to a hospital board (usually for an unspecified length of time) had appeared to be reserved for retired or semiretired citizens: people with "lots of idle time." Active, creative community citizens were often overlooked. Education and training for board members has never been stressed. Two problem areas result from this situation: (1) the board becomes heavily weighted with relatively inactive members, and (2) the management of the institution remains mystical and misunderstood and is left to the physicians and administration. Each board member is individual in interests, abilities, and willingness to invest time and effort in the position. Because an individual's priorities will change over time, it is important to identify lengths of terms so membership can be rotated regularly, drawing in new ideas and fresh enthusiasm.

Changing times

At times, trustees have not recognized the heavy responsibility of hospital board membership and have not been committed to the institution they represent. This has prompted the development of certain guidelines, and in some instances, even laws for hospital trustees. In Michigan, for instance, the legislature has established enforceable standards that apply to hospital trustees: "The governing body of each hospital shall be responsible for: . . . the operation of the hospital; . . . the selection of the medical staff; . . . the quality of care rendered in the hospital."[2]

Several strategic shifts, either afoot or needed, are changing or will change the composition, performance, and capabilities of the board. The changes primarily have to do with the age, training, and expertise of board members. In this vein, a contemporary development strategy of prime importance for boards of trustees/directors includes the following:

1. Board member training in terms of their roles, skills, and knowledge for that institution
2. Examination of various models for organizing boards and then designing and putting into operation one that fits
3. Building boards of trustees' goals and responsibilities that are board specific
4. Defining the requirements, rules, and processes for its own succession
5. Determining the appropriate size and mix of the board in terms of proportions of outside and inside directors.

Some recommendations

If it is agreed that boards of trustees/directors can have a significant impact on a hospital and its future, some recommendations aimed at maximizing the board's contributions are in order.

Boards of trustees should be trained and skilled in interpersonal relations because they have intimate contact with many groups within the institution and the community as well as with various representatives of the media. How a board member articulates the causes and concerns of the board of trustees may make the difference between cooperation and opposition on a pertinent issue. Board membership should be solicited from those who will essentially make a second career of their board activities and who will regularly devote time to hospital affairs.

An important aspect that should be addressed by each governing board and its sponsoring body is the appropriate size and composition of its membership. A hospital board should be somewhat representative of its constituency. It is important to have variety in its membership—in education, philosophy, experience, expertise, politics, religion, race, sex, and age. A board made up of a cross section of the community the hospital serves will increase the likelihood of meeting community needs and fostering community involvement. It is worthwhile for a board to occasionally inventory itself for such necessary skills as management, finance, planning, public relations, production, and marketing. The management of a health care institution is a complex business; its governing board should represent this same complexity.

Because the board deals chiefly with the administrator and medical staff, a fundamental issue is lay versus expert authority. A good argument can be made for inclusion on the board of those who are most intimately familiar with the operation of the facility, that is, physicians, nurses, and administrative leaders.

There is a recent move in hospitals, especially those operating for a profit, to appoint more physicians to boards of trustees. Twenty years ago, physicians on hospital boards were rare. Where physicians were appointed, the board usually contained no more than a "token" representative. By contrast, recent studies[4] have shown that more than half of all boards now include physicians.

If one subscribes to the philosophy that the physician is the customer of the hospital, then it is easy to understand the reasons for and objectives in encouraging greater physician participation on governing boards. One of the most pressing problems is spiraling hospital costs. Because quality and cost-of-care decisions are inseparable, management and governing boards must include the patient's purchaser of services—the physician—in the deliberations. Only in this manner can fundamental changes be made or effective controls developed.

A second and equally important reason for including physicians on the governing board was established in the legal principle affirmed in the *Charleston* case (*Darling*), that the hospital board is responsible for the quality of professional care provided by the institution. Hospitals and boards of trustees are legally required to maintain a medical staff structure that recommends and develops professional standards of care and that ensures the enforcement of these standards. Physicians are the obvious experts.

Greater public scrutiny, increased third-party interest in reimbursement procedures, and greater federal and state involvement provide additional justification for increased physician representation on boards. When accountability is addressed, it is best to have on the board a representative who is intimately familiar with those services for which the hospital is being held accountable. This consideration further justifies the inclusion of nurses and administrators on the board. Within these two groups lies the greatest knowledge of the operations of the financial and patient care components of the hospital. It is generally conceded that there is need for changes in the delivery of health care and in researching and developing new and innovative schemes for delivery emphasizing prevention. To effect even the most minor of these changes will require participation by all providers. Physicians, nurses, and administrators can help to shape the process.

It is plausible to assume that the number of members on the governing board of a hospital, together with their backgrounds, will have a substantial impact on the hospital's ability to respond to day-to-day problems and long-term issues. Although there is little evidence that relates board size, composition, or policies to board effectiveness or hospital performance,[15] a board better prepared to deal with any given problem should lead to better performance. Conversely, inactive, unresponsive boards retard both services and growth of the institution. Boards in conflict cause community rifts, which decrease hospital effectiveness, image, prestige, and the bottom line. Criteria that boards of trustees/directors might consider in assessing themselves are presented here:

1. Membership
   Is it representative?
   Does it reflect a variety of skills, opinions, ideas?
   Are all members active?
2. Purpose
   What are the goals?
   How is success measured?
   Are roles and responsibilities clear?
   Have all board members had an adequate orientation to board membership?
   What is the board's response to hospital employees?
   Are community needs and expectations being met?
3. Group development
   What is the feeling-tone of the meetings?
   Does everyone feel free to contribute?
   Are issues adequately discussed?
   Are power issues interfering with effective decision making?
   How cogent are members' interpersonal and communication skills?
4. Awareness
   Is the board open to community input?
   Is the board responsive to hospital employees?
   Is data gathering ongoing and perceived as everyone's task?

For the most part, the problems of the hospital addressed by the board of directors are not susceptible to easy, short-term, or indeed any permanent solutions. The nurse recruitment-retention dilemma that faces most hospitals today is a perfect example of the kind of problem that has no easy answer. In fact, many other problems with which the board member must deal can have their origins in the basic retention dilemma: unionization of health care workers, closing of hospital beds (especially in critical care areas), increases in cost per patient day, and so on. The dissatisfaction among consumers of health care today is unmistakeable, and a major cause tends to be hospital costs and policies. Pressure is exerted by consumers, taxpayers, and governmental agencies on the one hand, and personnel, managers, and medical staff on the other.

The assessment described above, followed by development and change (perhaps with the help of an organizational development/process consultant) can promote a board of trustees that has an understanding of the complexity of issues and an ability to deal with them. Such a group is prepared to work, understands interdependence, works for long-term resolution, and values institutional health. All of these are characteristics necessary to confront the retention issue in today's hospitals. The recommendations are intended to be those that will most positively affect the entire institution and its long-range operation.

In addition, there are other strategies and suggestions that will positively affect the *specific* problem of nurse turnover:

1. A nurse (perhaps the top-ranking nurse executive of that facility) should be included on the board of trustees. Some for-profit groups include on the board a vice-president of nursing. The same board-level membership could be accorded the top nursing executive in a not-for-profit hospital.
2. A board subcommittee should be created whose primary responsibility is nursing—to be updated, informed, and hospital-specific. This committee should be aware of turnover-retention statistics and how the hospital ranks within the community, state, and nation.

Most of the foregoing suggestions and recommendations have been tried on a piecemeal basis at various hospitals across the country. An individual hospital that wishes to create and support a milieu that facilitates retention needs to institute more than piecemeal, token changes. A comprehensive commitment for organization health is mandatory, beginning with the board. Any attempt to address the nationwide shortage of nursing (i.e., nursing retention) must include large-scale implementation of these and other proactive strategies.

HOSPITAL ADMINISTRATOR

The role and function of the hospital chief executive officer (CEO) or administrator is one of the most challenging in the business world. Administrators function in settings ranging from small community or specialty hospitals of 50 to 100 beds to large teaching hospitals or regional medical centers of over 1000 beds. Differences in settings necessitate different administrative behaviors. Whereas the administrator of a small hospital may know the names of all the hospital employees, the CEO of a large institution may know the names of few other employees besides the administrative staff. Because of the dynamic environment and the technological, political, economic, and social changes that have occurred in the past two decades, the CEO position of a hospital has become a highly diversified role. The role requires that the individual meet expectations that are imposed by a number of groups (board of trustees, medical staff, employees, government, community, etc.). The behavior of the administrator varies considerably depending on the nature of the group, the actual or perceived power of the group, the current publicity of the group's cause, and the amicability between the group and the administrator.

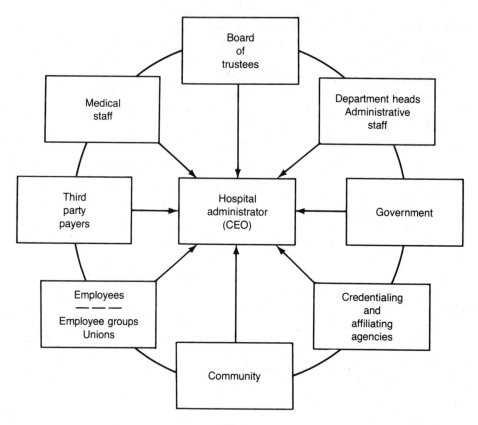

FIG. 6-2
Role and responsibility forces confronting the CEO.

A summary of the many groups impinging on the authority of the administrator is depicted graphically in Fig. 6-2.

Given the complexity of the environment, the manager (administrator) is almost required to have a graduate degree in hospital administration (MHA) or in business administration (MBA). Today's CEOs need skills different from those needed by their predecessors in the 1960s. Among the skills most essential for the CEO are marketing and planning.

Marketing

It has seemed crass to think of "marketing" a hospital and its services when we normally think of marketing in terms of selling detergent, automobiles, or food. Yet marketing is a critical issue among hospitals because of pressures to maintain old sources and find new sources of income. The old sources—government, insurance companies, and patients—are becoming more resistant, demanding justification and accountability for services and charges. In order to run the business more responsively and responsibly, hospital administrators are turning to new ideas and new services and are trying to sell them to the community. Marketing has become a necessary tool for developing viable programs and increasing public awareness of the hospital's services.

There is growing awareness among hospital administrators, boards, and physicians that hospitals must compete to survive. Marketing can be an important tool. Three target groups that can be influenced by aggressive marketing techniques are as follows:

1. Consumers: A large percentage of the hospital patient population chooses its hospital.
2. Physicians: Success with attached clinic buildings and lower cost malpractice insurance indicate physicians feel some loyalty toward hospitals they perceive as being interested in their well-being.
3. Nurses: Nurses' willingness to work at a hospital affects that hospital's ability to operate all of its beds. Nurses choose to work or not to work, and probably more important, where to work in the community. References such as Cooper's *Health Care Marketing: Issues and Trends*[4] provide basic information on some successful health care marketing endeavors.

Strategy formulation and strategic planning

There is a compelling need for the CEO of a hospital to initiate strategic and long-range planning. Strategic planning focuses on specific products and services and their fit with the long-range mission of the institution. Such planning requires a change in thinking from facility-oriented master planning to market-oriented strategic planning.

The key to successful strategic planning is the active involvement of the hospital's key personnel so that each has commitment to the final plan. In addition, the administrator must build a support group outside of the hospital made up of representatives from all constituencies who may be influenced by the strategic plan. By carefully building commitment inside and outside the hospital, the administrator can be more assured of the support needed to allocate and reallocate resources to initiate new projects and to cease antiquated programs.

After an institutional plan, either marketing or strategic, has been developed and approved by appropriate constituents, the timing and critical path to accomplish the plan largely rests with the CEO. This is done with the development and implementation of policies and planning for change.

One of the hallmarks of an effective organization—reflective of the CEO's ability to implement change—is his or her willingness to include executive and middle management staff in the planning and implementing of change. No management person can support what he or she does not understand, nor can commitment be expected. It is this middle management level that is so crucial in effective communication to all hospital employees.

More often than not, change requires cooperation. Management team members led by the CEO have the responsibility to gain support and cooperation to ensure a smooth and timely transition from the old to the new. It is also important to acknowledge that employees may react to change with resistance. Understanding and preparing for this resistance as a part of the change process will enable it to be dealt with in a positive manner (see Chapter 8).

Feedback must be incorporated into every component of the CEO's role. It is through this mechanism that effective evaluation of "performance to plan" is carried out. At critical points the CEO must respond to feedback received in order to continue the uninterrupted feedback mechanism. Each step must be carefully assessed in a timely manner and all implications must be considered. Feedback is not evaluative. Rather, it is focused on specific behavior and results, not on qualities of persons. Feedback is possible only when the person providing it believes he or she can be frank and honest *and* believes the feedback will be valued. When what is desired on the output side is not being achieved, the CEO has the responsibility to make adjustments. In order to bring about change, evaluation must be an ongoing process rather than an annual exercise.

The requisite skills that a CEO needs to be successful have an analogy in the nursing process: assessment, planning, implementation, evaluation—terms that are familiar to nurses at all levels and in all roles. The way in which a CEO uses these skills as a part of the administrative role can support and positively impact on the way nurses practice their use of this process in their job setting. The extent to which nurses are rewarded, recognized for their contribution to patient care, and included in the decision-making process will determine how successful the institution is in managing nurse retention, morale, and productivity.

Many hospital administrators see in their mind's eye the corporation president as the preferred organizational model. The title of administrator is being replaced by president in some not-for-profit institutions (as well as in for-profit hospitals), as they expand their role and scope to gain advantages enjoyed by the for-profit chains.

Depending on whether the institution is chartered as for profit or not for profit, there are greater or fewer differences between the corporate executive and the hospital executive. In a hospital owned by a for-profit corporation, the performance of the chief executive can be measured in much the same way as for a counterpart in any other service business. The CEO in either setting is held accountable for the year's results as quantified by net profit, contribution to return on investment, and earnings per share of the parent corporation. Such measurements cannot be made with as much validity or accuracy in a not-for-profit setting.

Any hospital administrator's successes are difficult to quantify or to analyze but the results are nonetheless apparent: (1) a financially sound institution, (2) productivity levels consistent with established standards, (3) consistently high levels of quality of care as evidenced by positive patient questionnaires and market surveys, and (4) a quality assurance program that has minimized risk exposure for the institution.

The successful CEO of the future will probably not be the one with visions of a new building addition or expansionary program. The new CEO must deal with increased regulations, competition, national health insurance in some form, increasing complexity of hospitals and services, more technological innovations, costs that continue to increase, expanding demand for outpatient services, and hospitals that will increasingly be a part of integrated systems. There must be a philosophical change in thinking by the CEO, from "more is better" to the realization that perhaps success can best be measured by the ability to contract strategically rather than expand; to eliminate rather than duplicate; and to merge rather than diversify. All of these will be accomplished by careful strategic planning, collaboration, negotiation, and creativity.

HOSPITAL MANAGEMENT

The past two decades have been noteworthy for the development and growth of health institutions based on corporate models. Traditionally the delivery system of health care institutions has consisted of clinics, private and public nonprofit voluntary hospitals, proprietary hospitals, teaching and research institutions, and extended care and rehabilitation facilities. Many of these institutions are finding it difficult to exist autonomously and have sought some type of affiliation with other institutions or groups, ranging on a continuum from total merger to shared services such as purchasing or laundry. The types of organizing and financing that hospitals are using include merger, joint venture, holding-company concept, investor-owned national hospital companies, and management contracts. The hospital under the direction of a multihospital management company "appears to have achieved a measure of efficiency and productivity not seen in the not-for-profit sector."[17] There is, however, a great deal of disagreement on what type of organizational structure is best. None has a clearly provable edge.

There are many alternative ways to classify hospitals, such as by size or specialty, but probably no classification scheme is more misleading or misunderstood than that of for profit versus not for profit. Regardless of its classification, no hospital can be a truly "charitable" institution; it cannot give its services away if it expects to keep its doors open and stay in business.

> All managers have, logically and morally, a "surplus" goal—to operate as managers so that the group for which they are responsible will achieve whatever the purpose or objectives may be with the minimum of expenditure of human and material resources or to achieve as much of a purpose as possible with the resources at their command.[10]

Thus the term *not for profit* does not connote "nonprofit" or "without charge." It is the source of the income and destination of the outgo that distinguishes for-profit from not-for-profit hospitals.

Not for profit

Voluntary or not-for-profit hospitals receive their initial funding from bond issues, from donations, or—in the case of federal, state, and county facilities—from governmental appropriations. By operating, they generate monies from the sale of hospital services. The income is used for the following:
- Facility expansion and facility debt retirement
- Salaries and benefits
- Repairs and renovation
- New capital equipment and retirement of debt on existing equipment

Additional monies for expansion or large projects may come only from the sale of more bonds, a major fund drive, or a plea to the appropriate government for more tax money.

For profit

Proprietary or for-profit hospital corporations receive their initial funding from the sale of stock just as in any other corporation. In the same manner as not-for-profit hospitals, their continued operation is funded by income from the sale of services. The income is used for the same purposes as for a not-for-profit hospital, with the addition of the following:
- Contribution to corporate management
- Taxes
- Stockholder dividends

Lack of profit (loss) at one hospital in a chain may be offset by profits at another. Additional large sums of money for expansion may be generated through the sale of more stock.

Recognizing their inherent disadvantage when it comes to generating expansion monies, many of the not-for-profit stand-alone hospitals are entering other ventures and forming associations for sharing such items as purchasing and computer facilities. Thus even the fiscal lines of delineation blur when differentiating between for-profit and not-for-profit hospitals.

With methods of operation becoming increasingly similar, hospitals must also have equivalent personnel procedures and salaries, organization designs, and management styles to survive. More importantly for the subject of this book, neither sector can depend on personal commitment to nursing to keep staff nurses on the job. Bold and substantial action taking in each of these three areas—directed toward nurses—is the critical "next step" for hospital management groups vis-à-vis nurse retention.

NURSING ADMINISTRATOR

The leader of the nursing department of a hospital may have any one of many titles and play a major or minor part in the decision making and management of the institution depending on his or her initiative and motivation, the attitude of the hospital administrator, and the organizational structure. The part played by nursing in decision making is dependent on the director at least as much as on the beliefs and values of the administrator and the institution's defined relationships. Because nursing usually makes up 50% to 70% of the employees of the hospital and accounts for about 40% to 50% of the annual salary budget, it seems logical that the nursing administrator be a powerful figure in the hospital hierarchy. This is not always the case. Directors of nursing who are granted full partnership in the management of the institution through title, authority, responsibility, and appropriate remuneration are uncommon.

It is often by default that the director of nursing fails to occupy a more influential position in the hospital. Through failure to assert themselves, directors of nursing are frequently relegated to minor and low-power positions in the organizational hierarchy. A primary reason for a lack of confidence in their ability to compete, be heard, and win in the board rooms of our health care institutions frequently stems from having little or no formal preparation in nursing administration or in management.

In 1977, only 27% of nursing directors held a master's degree and an additional 24% were baccalaureate prepared.[14] The remaining 49% were graduates of 3-year diploma programs or 2-year associate degree programs—programs that include at best no more than a cursory introduction to leadership, and certainly no training for managing a major division of a large business.

Nurses are still promoted to fill vacancies because they are clinically competent or have seniority on the nursing administrative staff. Much of nursing leadership is learned by intuition, hit or miss, or imitation of a mentor no better educated than themselves.

Many nursing service administrators are entrenched in a bureaucratic system and do not have the skills, knowledge, or personal courage and fortitude to break out. Although nursing educators today are teaching their students about creativity, autonomy, and the ability to be a change agent, nursing directors and their management staff are still rewarding compliance and conformity and are fostering their own authority.

It is relevant commentary on nursing's past and its potential for future progress that nurses have never been able to unite on any issue. Nursing stands divided on every issue: what nursing is and does, what should be the basic preparation for the registered nurse, how nursing should relate to other disciplines, and who should manage nursing. Is it any wonder, even with practitioners numbering between one and two million, that nursing, divided, is not a threat to anyone?

Staff nurses in hospitals feel strongly that their directors must have and exercise influence in the institutions for them to receive recognition and job satisfaction. This cannot occur with a director who is unable to work cooperatively with the administration and medical staff and who is unable to bring the nursing staff's input into the formation and implementation of patient care standards.

Nursing directors too often continue to maintain the status quo, aligning themselves with hospital administration and the medical staff. By so doing, they shirk their responsibilities of team building and unification of nurses to improve the practice of hospital nursing. Nurses must receive recognition for a job well done. They need a leader who can rejoice with them in a sense of accomplishment and achievement and help them to receive satisfaction from the work they do. With such a director, nurses will begin to realize higher levels of personal growth and rewards for the practice of nursing, and hospital nursing will become a desirable job setting. Only then will professional nurses be retained.

In addition to the issue of job satisfaction, there is likely to be no end to the shortage of hospital nurses unless serious attention is given to the *economic* rewards of hospital nursing. The income of nurses during the past two decades has increased at a low rate. Their depressed income is a major factor in the current shortage of hospital nurses. As long as a nurse can secure a position requiring little investment (either in education or responsibility), in a nonemotionally charged environment, for the same or greater pay, there will be little incentive to remain in the nursing profession. In addition to the direct monetary benefit seen in the paycheck, administration can provide conditions that have the effect of increased salary. Some of these are described in Chapter 2 on recruitment. In general, a willingness to accommodate nurses' individual situations at one hospital may offset an apparently higher salary structure at another.

It is the director of nursing who sets the pace and creates the climate for nursing practice. It is this atmosphere that is so important in retaining nursing staff. The best indication of real morale in an institution is for a nurse to ask a colleague, "Why don't you come to work at the hospital where I work?" If a nurse feels uncomfortable being such an unofficial recruiter, it is incumbent on the nursing director to determine the reason and to change conditions. The best recruiters for nursing staff in an institution are employees and former patients, but the best retainers of these nurses once recruited are nursing managers led by the director of nursing.

INTERDEPARTMENTAL RELATIONS

Nursing, by the nature of its role and 24-hour responsibility to patient care, influences and is influenced by many other departments within the hospital. Among the departments most affected by nursing are laboratory, radiology, pharmacy, dietary, admitting, materials management, and engineering.

Interdepartmental relations among nursing and these departments greatly affect the smooth performance of patient care and influence the nurse's care plan for the patient. The amount of support and cooperation that is perceived as necessary on both sides is a major element in these relationships. Too often, departmental interests compete and take precedence over quality patient care. It has become a battleground in some institutions as more tasks that are required on the evening (3 to 11) and night (11 to 7) shifts and on weekends are relegated to nursing because the ancillary departments close or operate with skeleton staffs. Frequently these supporting departments employ transporters to transport patients to and from tests during the week, but on weekends the department has no transporter and nurses are asked to provide this service. Because nurses are directly responsible for the care patients receive, it seems fitting that they request and deploy support services. In actuality, they have no authority to redirect the resources of the hospital to carry out the duties expected of them. As long as the support staff remains inadequate in number, nurses, as the only 24-hour professional caregivers, will continue to have to assign nursing personnel from direct care to support services.

A few minutes' thought will verify that nursing provides services that could more efficiently be carried out by the support departments. The reasons may be inadequate personnel within ancillary departments or abdication of responsibilities by those departments. For whatever reason, many services provided by nursing, particularly on the night shift, should be under the cognizance of the following departments:

- Housekeeping
- Pharmacy
- Radiology

- Admitting/business office
- Dietary
- Laboratory
- Engineering
- Materials management

Examples of the duties carried out by nurses that fall in each of these departments are shown below. Considering the wide range of services expected of nurses and provided by them (perhaps by default), considering their lack of formal authority to carry out the responsibilities heaped upon them, and considering their lack of recognition for being able to carry out the tasks at all (let

---

INEFFICIENT USES OF NURSING RESOURCES

HOUSEKEEPING

Making unoccupied beds
Delivering fresh water, cleaning water pitchers
Mopping floors in OR and delivery suites especially on the evening and night shifts
Cleaning spills and patient excreta from floors on evening and night shifts
Defrosting and cleaning refrigerators and ice machines on patient units
Emptying trash and lining containers on evening and night shifts
Cleaning utility rooms and nursing stations
Stripping beds after patient discharge
Cleaning equipment on patient units

ENGINEERING

Doing preventive maintenance on equipment
Reporting problems without appropriate reaction or remedy, so nurses attempt repair

ADMITTING AND BUSINESS OFFICE

Transporting patients
Explaining room charges to patients
Answering insurance questions
Coordinating room assignments for patients

MATERIALS MANAGEMENT

Getting supplies after hours
Counting carts
Checking sterility dates
Making charges, validating shortages
Contacting manufacturers' representatives concerning problems
Requesting supplies with no feedback regarding request

DIETARY

Delivering meals and snacks
Checking to ensure that patients receive prescribed diet

alone well), is it any wonder hospitals have difficulty keeping nurses on staff and productive?

The degree to which nursing has to assume responsibilities that should have been relegated to support services depends on the size of the institution and the philosophy of the administrator and director of nursing. If administration creates a climate where all departments are provided with personnel support adequate to carry out their services during the hours they are needed, the benefits will cascade downward to nursing. Such a philosophy set by top administration is supported and perpetuated by department heads. In hospitals where this philosophy prevails, ancillary department heads will provide

---

DIETARY—cont'd

Making trips to dietary to obtain late trays for patients or items omitted from trays

Removing empty trays from patients' rooms

Distributing and collecting menus

Rotating nourishment stock in unit refrigerator

PHARMACY

Dispensing medications from pharmacy on evening and night shifts and on weekends

Making trips to pharmacy to obtain drugs for stat doses and to start newly ordered medications

Making medicine cart counts

Mixing patient intravenous fluids

Giving instructions to patients regarding medications

LABORATORY/RADIOLOGY

Having to carry requisitions or specimens for tests to laboratory

Having to transport patients to X-ray department for exams when they do not have this service available

Scheduling tests when no one is in department

Making arrangements for patients to be sent elsewhere when equipment is out of service

Returning films to X-ray department and retrieving films for X-ray

CLERICAL/UNIT MANAGEMENT

Having to transcribe data, which is time consuming and better handled by a clerical person

Ordering supplies to stock units

Following up shortages on supplies

Taking minutes in staff meetings

Typing records and forms

Coordinating pilot projects requested by other departments

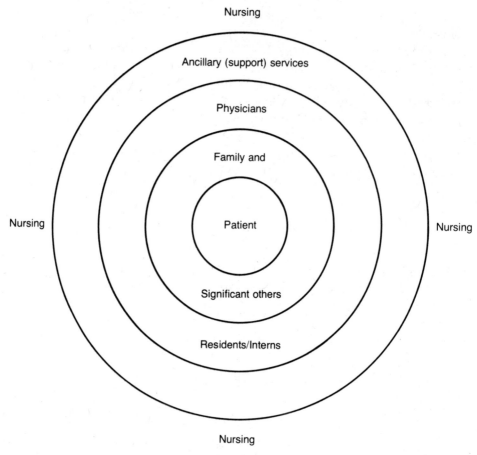

FIG. 6-3
Nursing: coordinators of caregivers.

their services in order to free nurses to provide more direct patient care. The bottom line will be that nurses will be able to do their job better, feel more kindly and less frustrated toward themselves, and stay on the job rather than pursuing the pot of gold from one hospital to the next.

Regardless of the philosophy and support of administration, nurses will remain the coordinators of all caregiving (see Fig. 6-3). This role is charged with 24-hour responsibility for assuring continuity of patient care and for preventing fragmented or incomplete care. An organization cannot hope to solve the long-term nurse retention problem unless in its basic philosophy it understands the role of the professional nurse and values the unique contribution that nurses make and have to make to patient care.

COLLEGIALITY WITH PHYSICIANS

A sensitive area with nurse managers and staff nurses alike is their per-ceived lack of status in the hospital hierarchy. It should be noted that this perception is organizationwide. Nurses in the past have been looked on as combinations of gofers and handmaidens, with the pay and respect usually ac-corded these two groups. Physicians accord no one equality. Many feel it their prerogative to berate nurses in front of their peers and coworkers for perceived infractions in carrying out treatment orders. The nurses, recogniz-ing they are being accorded much less than equal status, may react in any one of several ways:

- They may retreat, trying to do no more than they are "ordered" to do by the physicians, and doing as they are ordered even if they believe it to be incorrect. Such action, of course, results in an even further deteriora-tion of nurses' feelings of self-esteem.
- They may try to meet the physician head-on, arguing toe-to-toe in an attempt to force concessions and demand respect from the physician. This has the result of further undermining the relationship between two groups who should be cooperating and complementary.
- They may attempt to follow the chain of command and work through the hospital administration to improve conditions. This course of action is usually not fruitful unless there is a very strong hospital administrator. In addition, it may be seen by physicians as a symptom of nurses' weak-ness and unwillingness to confront the problem head-on (i.e., face-to-face with the physicians).

A close look at each of the three situations above reveals that the nurse is placed in a no-win position. No matter what the nurse's action, the reaction is generally that of reinforcing the already stereotyped image of the nurse as "unprofessional" or "pushy."

The solution to the problem of the nursing profession's lack of status lies not in isolated effort on the part of nurses, but instead in a concerted effort toward progress through organizational change by the entire hospital.

One hospital executive says: "There are almost always special require-ments for progress. Frequently there must be some catalyst for develop-ment."[7] The catalyst for development of a better professional relationship between physicians and nurses will have to come from nurses and will re-quire a philosophical change on the part of the physician. Nursing is not a service for the physician; rather it is a service for patients. This philosophy is given lip service in our institutions but nurses experience a reality that is different. The nurse-physician relationship is the most tenuous in all of health care. The collaborative practice model that is so desperately needed in our health care institutions has not been fully developed or implemented; in many cases it is not even considered. The model depicted in Fig. 6-4 requires

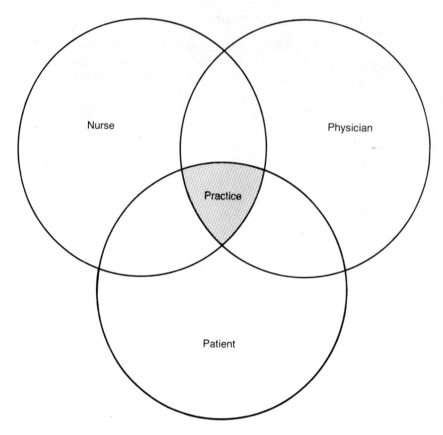

FIG. 6-4
A model of current nurse-physician collaboration.

the professional knowledge and skills of the nurses and physicians to come together on at least a quasi-equal level to have a maximum favorable impact on the patient's health.

Physicians do not fully understand the role of the nurse in health care and many do not feel that the development of an interdisciplinary team approach or collaborative practice in patient care is needed. They fear that it will interfere with the practice of their profession.

Nurses have over the years desired to work as colleagues with physicians in hospitals, but the mechanism to make this happen has yet to be discovered. Nurses often doubt their contributions and question their roles in relation to physicians, contributing to frustration, disillusionment, and disappointment with the profession. In nursing schools, nursing students are taught autonomy, responsibility, and critical thinking. As graduates they find their role somewhere between handmaiden and executive secretary, but always in a master-servant relationship with physicians. This disparity between the way things could be and the way they actually are has caused many competent, caring nurses to leave hospitals, never to return.

Physicians, in turn, have gaps in their training when it comes to working relationships. Advisement and instruction are given in developing a bedside manner, but in general none is given toward developing rapport with one's colleagues (except possibly the physician fraternity). This leads to management by imitation, with the younger physicians miming the behavior of their more experienced peers. Invariably, the learned style is autocratic, with the nurse being the subordinate in the nurse-physician relationship.

Some of nursing's most difficult problems to overcome are found in relationships. There are fundamental incompatibilities in contractual and implied relationships among physicians, hospitals, and professional nurses. The difficulties encountered by nurses in their professional role are in the following areas of authority:

I. Clinical decision making: Because of their formal training and experience, nurses should be recognized and heeded as valuable resources in the gathering of information to make clinical decisions and in the making of decisions in areas of their expertise.
   A. Problems are encountered in setting up formal and informal two-way communication between physicians and nurses relating to the care of a particular group of patients.
   B. Formation of and acceptance in a joint practice committee should be a goal.
   C. Joint evaluation of patient care should be based on established standards developed by physicians and nurses.
   D. Physicians and supervisors should accept clinical judgments that are within acceptable standards of nursing practice and made using medical-nursing consultations.
   E. Nurses make decisions to start or discontinue treatments that are appropriate to protocol and standards.
II. Technology applications: The nurse should be able to initiate the application or removal of certain technological equipment or special services.
   A. Weaning patient from ventilators
   B. Nutritional support consultations
   C. Monitoring of cardiac status by telemetry
   D. Moving patient to critical care areas when indicated
III. Nursing diagnosis and orders
   A. Nursing interventions based on nursing diagnosis and orders should be recognized by third-party payers as legitimate and reimburseable.
   B. Physicians and hospital administration should recognize nursing orders as an integral part of the patient care plan.

IV. Coordinator of all caregivers: The nurse with 24-hour responsibility has to have the ultimate authority in the coordination of care and support services for a group of designated patients.
   A. Primary nursing embraces this concept.
   B. Interdisciplinary committees and support groups are organized to solve problems and implement change.
   C. Nurses must have sufficient authority in their work setting to make decisions and apply technology as they accept responsibility for their professional practice.

It is going to be difficult to change more than a century of traditional nurse-physician relationships and the change will be traumatic both for physicians and nurses. This change involves a complete rethinking of nurse-physician roles, responsibilities, and accountability for patient care. The implications of this change process for the future of nurse retention in hospitals are positive. However, until physicians are willing to work with nurses and hospital administration to foster participation by nurses in organizational decision making, the vital collegial relationships will never come to fruition. And until nurses personally and individually demonstrate their worth and strengths in patient care, and their managerial skill and knowledge, physicians will not be prompted to foster such participation. Nurses must take these *interpersonal risks* to attain the professional status they deserve.

ORGANIZATIONAL STRUCTURES AND POLICIES
Role theory and role functions

The *formal* organizational structure within a group has a great deal to do with how people act and react, what they perceive their roles to be, how others perceive them, how well and in what direction(s) information flows, and, ultimately, how much cooperation and coordination exists among those people. The act of formalizing the structure by publishing an organization chart provides much information to employees about authority-responsibility relationships, what roles are played by the participants, the influence each role has, and directions of communication flow. This formal structure is further defined and confined by the rules, policies, and procedures made up and published by the committee in the governance structure.

The nurse's place in the formal organizational structure, when coupled with his or her *perceived* place or role as a caregiver, have led to severe role conflicts. The root of such conflicts can perhaps be traced back to nurses' training. In many cases, the student nurse is expected to be in a subservient position, not questioning the information imparted but instead absorbing it. Whether in the lecture hall or on the floor, it is impressed upon the student nurse that he or she is the *student* and not an equal or near-equal partner in patient care. (To be fair, it must be stated that such is the case in most other

college and university training programs as well.) From here the graduate
nurse goes to a position as a "new" nurse who must confront

- A new organization, with new policies, procedures, methods, and standards of care
- A new nurse supervisor, usually trained in a different school and doubt-
  less with different ideas on how care on the unit should be administered
- A new group of physicians who likely see the new nurse as fertile
  ground for further training in their own methods of health care, including preferred procedures

Assuming the above conditions have accuracy, is it reasonable to expect
the nurse suddenly to blossom and to negotiate/earn a quasi-equal position
with the physician on the patient care team? Is it reasonable to assume the
nurse can fundamentally change his or her role in the hospital? It is extremely
unlikely that such will be the case. A better way to describe why the above
change in nurse attitude and role cannot occur spontaneously is to examine
the Lawrence and Lorsch model of behavior change in organizations.[11] According to their model (Fig. 6-5), changes required in the organization's behavior range from modest to fundamental. For each of the behavior changes to
occur, the preceding change must be in place and operational. This is haz-
ardous when one realizes that the successive changes involve greater emotional investment.

As an example, suppose a hospital makes a decision to do something
about the problem of high turnover. Suppose further that the "method" selected to address the problem is that of changing the attitudes or feelings of
the nurses about themselves (i.e., to make them feel more needed and more a
part of the patient care team).

1. For such a change to occur, there must be different interaction patterns
   between the physicians and nurses and between the staff and supervisory nurses.
2. In order for different interaction to become effective, the physicians
   and nurses must have role expectations that are different from those
   currently operational. That is, the physicians must *expect* the nurses to
   take on an equal (or near-equal) and valued role in the development
   and execution of a patient care plan. The nurses, in turn, must *expect
   to be expected* to do so. Notice here that the behavior changes are
   already becoming more fundamental than modest.
3. For the different roles and expectations discussed above to become
   realized, there must be a shift in orientation, values, and *valuing* on
   the part of the physicians, nurses, and nursing supervisors. Physicians
   must perceive nurses as being important caregivers with professional
   training, practical experience, invaluable opportunity to continuously

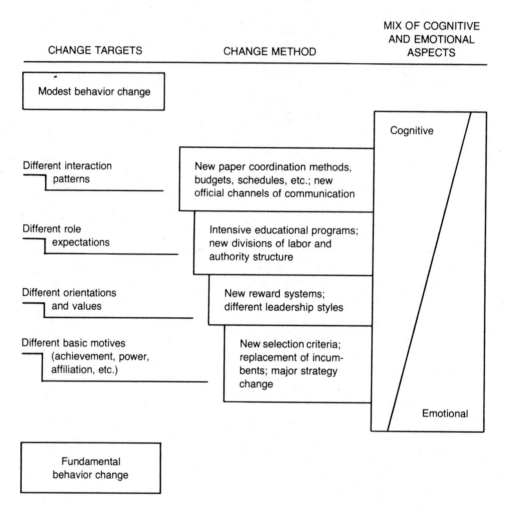

FIG. 6-5

Behavior change in organizations. (From Lawrence, P., and Lorsch, V.: Developing organizations: diagnosis and action, Reading, Mass., 1969, Addison-Wesley Publishing Co., Fig. 6. Reprinted with permission.)

observe the patients, and valuable opinions. For their part, the nurses and supervisors must perceive *themselves* as possessing these attributes. As noted in the model, this will necessitate a change in leadership styles on the part of both nurse supervisor and physician as well as a change in the follower style of the staff nurse. That is, it will necessitate the willingness of the staff nurse to accept such a leadership style and the responsibility inherent in being led in such a manner.

4. Finally, basic shifts in the orientation and values of the caregivers presuppose shifts in the basic motives of the health care organization.

Notice the change method suggested by the model. Notice also the relative cognitive/emotional mix for a change at this level.

Essentially, the previous discussion demonstrates the fact that a change in the health care organization necessary to bring about a fundamental change in the pattern of nurse retention must start at the board level and flow downward through the entire organizational structure. The board—the governing body of the entire institution—must change its strategy to one of recognizing the retention problem and confronting it. Such a strategy requires that the board address the organization structure and its design.

Designs and their implications

Many types of organization structure are possible within a health care organization. In essence, all are variations or combinations of two very basic structures: (1) functional organization and (2) product organization.

Functional organization. In a functional industrial organization, everyone devoted to carrying out a given *function* (e.g., finance) reports upward to the director of that function. Applied to nursing, all nurses report to the director or vice-president of nursing. Such a structure concentrates competence in effective ways and stimulates colleague interaction. It does deemphasize interdependency and cooperation, can create boundaries between departments, and inhibits lateral communication.

Product organization. The usual product organization has everyone concerned with building a given product or providing a given service reporting to the manager of that product or service. Applied to hospitals, everyone in the emergency department (ED) reports to the head of the ED. This structure allows for better intragroup communication and facilitates accountability, but it may pose problems in terms of job loyalties and professional stimulation.

A relatively recent addition to organization theory and practice is project team or matrix organization. A matrix organization consists of a hybrid of the function and product organizations. People are pulled from the various functional units needed to carry out a given project or task. Individual tasks often do not require full-time effort of team members. Thus each member may be on two or more teams at any given time. Each team member is responsible to the team leader for performance of his or her function on a particular team, while still reporting to a functional head. In the matrix organization, which has each team member or nurse reporting to multiple supervisors, the potential problems include anarchy, confusion, power struggles, and "groupitis." The positive aspects of this design include efficiency, flexibility, technical excellence, and provision for personal development. The major requirement of a matrix organization is a continuing emphasis on communication. Unfortunately, within the curriculums of most health care workers, there is no course or subject area that specifically addresses this requirement.

ORGANIZATIONAL CLIMATE

One major deterrent to the nurse's quest for greater professional respect and recognition in the hospital lies within the organizational structure itself and in its attendant climate. Traditionally, the organization of a production enterprise is a rigid hierarchy. The different levels of the hierarchy are not supposed to deal directly with one another, but are instead supposed to follow the "chain of command." Thus an employee in one branch of an organization is not supposed to correct or give orders to a person above or in another branch of the organization.

Consider the unique position in which the type of hierarchy and traditional relationships noted above put the staff nurse.

1. The nurse reports upward in the administrative hierarchy. Thus a typical chain of command might lead from staff nurse to head nurse to assistant director of nursing to director of nursing to assistant/associate administrator to administrator to board of directors/trustees. Depending on the area of the country, profit orientation of the hospital, and other factors, the titles and the levels in the hierarchy may differ. In general, however, there will be a large number of levels between the staff nurse and the top of the organization.
2. The physicians report upward in the medical hierarchy. From the individual physicians the hierarchy usually proceeds from physician to chief of service to chief of the medical staff to the board of directors/trustees.

Given these two points, it is readily apparent that:

1. The route from individual contributor to the top of the organization is much shorter for the physician than the nurse.
2. Because (1) is true, the implication is that the nurse is in a much lower level position and is subordinate to the physician.
3. Because (2) is true, the tendency is not to pay as much heed to and give less credence to the input of nurses as compared to physicians.

When dealing with organizational and attitudinal frustrations inherent in (1), (2), and (3) above, it is relatively easy for the nurse to become a "voluntary resignee" either actually or figuratively.

The organizational structure and policies in a health care institution, combined with the attending organizational climate, violate several principles of management. These include (1) unity of command, and (2) parity of authority and responsibility.

Unity of command

It is usually conceded that an employee should be responsible to and held accountable by only one supervisor. This is not true by any means of the work life of the staff nurse, who has, in fact, multiple supervisors to satisfy.

First, the nurse must satisfy an immediate supervisor. Second, virtually any physician having privileges and patients at the hospital feels able to correct the nurse's behavior relative to the physician's patients. This means, in essence, that the nurse has responsibility to any number of physicians with these "functional supervisors" changing from hour to hour and day to day and with each having a different set of "managerial" quirks.

One well-known result of having multiple supervisors is the possibility of conflicting instructions. With physicians at any hospital having come from different medical school and residency programs, such conflicting instructions are not only a possibility, but a great probability. A second result of lack of unity of command is ambiguous accountability. Questioning of responsibility by nurses can have repercussions, particularly in quality of care.

Parity of authority and responsibility

Another principle of management states that a person's responsibility for actions should be neither more nor less than that implied by the authority delegated. A nurse, even a "nonsupervisory" staff nurse, effectively supervises the carrying out of a health care plan for several patients. This involves overseeing the work of such people as LPNs, nurse assistants, other orienting RNs, and volunteers. In addition, the nurse must note such things as a need for housekeeping and maintenance services and somehow see that they are provided. A nurse who sees an example of inadequate or incompetent care by a physician is responsible for bringing it to someone's attention in such a way as not to endanger working relationships with physicians. This amounts to tremendous responsibility without the requisite authority to make changes or improvements readily. The above-listed people are under the scrutiny of the nurse, who can be chastised for failing to correct inappropriate behavior on their part. Yet a look at the organizational chart of any hospital will fail to show these people reporting to the nurse.

ORGANIZATIONAL ATTITUDE: A WILLINGNESS TO INVEST

In any organization desiring to make great changes for the better, there must be a pervasive willingness to *invest*. Money must be spent on change. It is inevitable and it is important. It is equally important, however, for the organization to be willing to make other investments for very innovative changes, not just for the sake of being innovative, but for the good of the institution and its mission.

Risk taking

No major change, organizational or otherwise, can come about without risk taking on the part of the person or group being changed. The change of an entire organizational structure is no exception. Any major change in an organization, and especially change in the structure itself, must begin at the top. A change of this magnitude will be known—accurately or inaccurately— throughout the organization. Coupled with the knowledge will be fear.

If a health care institution expects to accomplish a major change in organization structure, some actions are essential:

1. A method must be used to involve those people affected by the new structure. Whether this is done by soliciting opinions and suggestions from all employee groups as part of the planning process or keeping the groups posted on events as they develop, each person must feel involved in the change process.

2. Enough study must have gone into the change to be reasonably certain that the new organization structure will be mostly correct, and therefore no additional major changes will be immediately forthcoming. Minor changes will be needed to fine tune the structure, but changes at the board or vice-presidential level should not be anticipated. If this basic rule is violated, the appearance will be that top management is groping and searching for anything that will work. The result will be lost support on the part of the employee.

3. The upcoming change should be introduced in a positive sense, that is, it should be acknowledged and marketed as a positive step rather than a remedial effort. Although it may not be necessary to convey the change in all its details, personnel should be informed of all changes that will affect them.

4. Information should be disseminated well in advance of any changes. It is very disconcerting to read the morning paper and find that the organization to which you have dedicated yourself has made a major shift and you were not informed.

Any organizational change is a risk, but managers of that organization must be willing to take risks in order to affect the organization in a positive sense. These suggestions will neither eliminate risk nor convince a group to take risks, but they will minimize risks once a change decision has been reached.

Money

Any change in the status quo of an organization requires commitment to pay the price. Some of this price involves money. In days of inflation, increasing scrutiny of all aspects of health care, and much publicity about the increasing costs of such care, it takes a good deal of courage on the part of the governing body of a hospital to agree to pay the dollar price of significant change.

In the case of nurses, one of the significant changes that must occur is in the form of salary commensurate with professional responsibilities. Their professional and nonprofessional duties are now broad enough. Supporting nurses as suggested in this book would greatly reduce or eliminate the nonprofessional duties now required, and would expand and enhance their professional role. This change alone will likely necessitate salary increases, and as the field of nursing continues to move toward the requirement of a baccalaureate degree, the pressure for better pay will intensify.

As noted above, it will take a courageous governing board to push for salary improvements for a group of employees as large as that of nursing. Consider, however, the turnover cost figures discussed in the first chapter. Even with other factors remaining constant, a decrease in turnover will free a substantial amount of money for salary increases.

Refer also to the box listing inefficient use of nursing resources in this chapter (pp. 194-195). If nurses perform all these tasks, they have less time to give the professional care for which they are qualified. If, instead, proper support is given to nursing on all shifts, fewer nurses will be needed. More support personnel will be needed, but they should be available at lower costs. Thus it would appear that the money commitment of the board and the administrator will be mainly a commitment to reallocate money rather than find new money.

Innovation

In any organization, an attempt at innovation in structure invariably meets with certain attitudes on the part of the personnel involved.

- People are often skeptical because it is a *change*.
- It requires selling for the same reason.
- It can meet with hidden as well as open animosity.

Many of the comments made in the section on risk taking are also appropriate here. The reception given to an innovation by a work force is generally determined by whether it perceives the innovation to be good or bad. Many changes that are radical, in retrospect, have been successfully implemented in hospitals because adequate groundwork was laid throughout affected groups. Some of these innovative changes are discussed in Chapter 7.

In this chapter, the changes suggested in the hospital environment are based on planned change (see Chapter 8) and thus are global in nature. This is intentional and necessary. It is improbable for a series of isolated, fragmented departmental changes to bring about the transformation in atmosphere necessary to improve nurse retention. Instead, there must be a concerted, well-planned and executed, coordinated effort involving and affecting everyone from the board through the lowest echelon in the hierarchy. As illustrated in this chapter, the necessary steps include

- A realization and an admission that there is a problem in nurse retention

- A solicitation of input from the people involved with the problem and its ramifications
- A strategic plan for implementation of agreed-on changes, plus a marketing plan if one is appropriate

These steps will cause changes throughout the hospital as suggested and stated in the chapter.

1. Board membership will change to reflect discrete terms, creative members, newer techniques, and representation of caregivers.
2. Nursing management will change to reflect the newly recognized value of the staff nurse.
3. Nursing support services will be augmented to allow nurses to carry out the duties for which they are professionally trained.
4. Nurses' salaries will increase.
5. Nursing turnover will decrease.

REFERENCES AND ADDITIONAL READINGS

1. Aiken, L.H.: Nursing priorities of the 1980's: hospitals and nursing homes, Am. J. Nurs. **81**(2):324-330, Feb. 1981.
2. Bigelow, J.: The new look in hospital trustees, Trustee **22**:10, Jan. 1969.
3. Carter, K.A.: Managerial role development in the nursing supervisor, Superv. Nurse **11**(7):26-28, July 1980.
4. Cooper, P.D., editor: Health care marketing: issues and trends, Germantown, Md., 1979, Aspen Systems Corp.
5. 1981 Directory of investor-owned hospitals and hospital management companies, Washington, D.C., 1980, Federation of American Hospitals.
6. Gilmore, K., and Wheeler, J.R.: A national profile of governing boards, Hospitals **46**:105-107, Nov. 1, 1972.
7. Groner, P.: Viewpoint—evolution of nurse-education, Pensacola News Journal, Jan. 24, 1982, p. 17A.
8. Grubbs, J., Haden, J.E., and Myers, D.N.: Bringing the medical staff into hospital planning by sharing data, Hospitals **55**(2):73-76, Jan. 16, 1981.
9. Johnson, R.L.: The power broker—prototype of the hospital chief executive? HCM Rev. **3**(4):67, Fall 1978.
10. Koontz, H., and O'Donnel, C.: Management: a systems and contingency analysis of managerial functions, New York, 1976, McGraw-Hill Book Co.
11. Lawrence, P.R., and Lorsch, J.W.: Developing organizations: diagnosis and action, Reading, Mass., 1969, Addison-Wesley Publishing Co.
12. Longest, B.B.: The contemporary hospital chief executive officer, HCM Rev. **3**(2):43, Spring 1978.
13. McMillan, N.H.: Marketing: a tool that serves hospitals' survival instincts, Hospitals **55**(23):89-92, Nov. 16, 1981.
14. National Commission on Nursing: Initial report and preliminary recommendations, Chicago, 1981.
15. Rakich, J.S., and Darr, K.: Hospital organization and management: text and readings, ed. 2, New York, 1978, S.P. Medical and Scientific Books.
16. Ready, R.K., and Ranelli, F.E.: Strategic and non-strategic planning in hospitals, HCM Rev. **7**(4):27-38, Fall 1982.

17. Siafaca, E.: Investor-owned hospitals and their role in the changing U.S. health care system, New York, 1981, F and S Press.
18. Schulz, R., and Johnson, A.C.: Management of hospitals, New York, 1976, Mc-Graw-Hill Book Co.
19. Theme, Carl W.: Strategic planning has market orientation, Hospitals **53**(23): 57-60, Dec. 1, 1979.

7

INNOVATIONS

CAUTION
INTRODUCTION
AN INDEX OF INNOVATIONS, PRESENTED ALPHABETICALLY

CAUTION

The basic values and concepts espoused in this book, with supporting research and theory, are assessment, diagnosis, the "fit" between ideas and organizations, attention to process and climate in conjunction with activities, and preparation and planning. *It is therefore inappropriate for readers to turn to this chapter for "answers."* These suggestions can only be understood, applied, and successful if implemented within the total framework advocated by and considerations presented within this entire effort. *Planned retention* is a way of *being* as well as a series of strategies and innovations. Do not apply these ideas without first clarifying and assuring their contributions to your comprehensive organizational plan for retaining professional staff nurses, enhancing quality of working life, and improving organization well-being and productivity.

INTRODUCTION

Chapter 7 presents innovations that are relevant to the primary concern of this book: the retention of the professional staff nurse. The innovations are appropriate for organizational-structural, administrative, managerial, and personal application. They are not meant to preclude the extensive number of suggestions presented throughout the remainder of the book; readers are encouraged to review the book in depth for such inputs. Additionally, each innovation may be an old thought or a radical departure. Each innovation is briefly described and expanded on. There has been little attempt to describe specifically how to implement the innovation, as it must be honed to fit each organization. Most importantly, each organization, administrator, manager, and ordinary person must carefully examine the innovation and decide whether it is appropriate to their relevant needs and circumstances. Perhaps the innovation will not work; perhaps it will not work but a variation will; perhaps the innovation will not work but it will lead the system to creative alternatives or lateral thinking activities. The purpose of this chapter is also to encourage organizations and people to take risks, not to stay where they are. It provides grist for talking together—for *changing*. Chapter 8 then provides the readers with the knowledge, skills, and strategies that will assure successful changes in behalf of organizations, persons, and health care. Keep track of your innovations and share them with others; you have a lot of help to offer others.

AN INDEX OF INNOVATIONS, PRESENTED ALPHABETICALLY
Allow change

To survive, organizations must change. Organizations change as they mature; they change in their focus as maturation indicates different critical concerns and issues. This change is often seen as normal; it is even often called evolving. Change can be healthy if it is embraced. If change is seen as valuable, the tools and formalized network requisite for implementing appropriate activities are more likely to be in place within a system. Too often change regarding the organization, its environment, and its management is perceived as a threat. Most hospital facilities are already aware of what will convince their employees to stay—more specifically, their professional staff nurse. But for some reason they see changing as "giving in" rather than simply acting to keep staff members. Organizations must recognize the appropriateness of *changing to retain*. They must adopt an attitude that allows them to consider change as a viable strategy in the retention process. Organizations must also create the apparatus necessary for preparing and planning for change. Equally important is the creation of a committee with rotating membership whose major responsibility is to stay alert to the need for change. Ongoing observation and assessment are primary tasks for such groups. Change for change's sake is not helpful. Change for the sake of organization profitability and task accomplishment is imperative. Retaining professional staff nurses is one change that is a relevant objective for health care facilities. Exploring "How can we change to retain nurses?" is a fair and acceptable management task.

Become politically astute

Health care is political fastball. Controls, regulations, accountability are expensive and far-reaching issues for health care in general as well as for nursing specifically. For most of their history, health care and health care-givers have naively gone about caring for the sick. Accusations that they have been inefficient, financially negligent, and noncircumspect in building are and were true. Rapid changes in the socioecopolitical structure of the day have made it suicidal for hospital administrators and nursing leaders to remain politically ignorant or inactive.

Davis and colleagues[4] have identified relevant issues and methods for the political novice that include (1) staying informed, (2) building a support base, and (3) providing directions. They further noted *basic* activities for effective interaction with political leaders. These are presented on p. 213.

Be professional

What formula ensures that nurses think and act professionally? There is no quick fix, no magic potion to effect the nonprofessional to professional transition. The fundamental responsibility must rest with the individual nurse in the commitment to nursing. It is personal acceptance of accountability for one's professional demeanor, behavior, performance, and image that the nurse wishes to convey to her colleagues and the public. The second area of responsibility for thinking and acting professionally is centered in the man-

---

THE BASIC ACTIVITIES
OF AN EFFECTIVE GOVERNMENT RELATIONS OPERATION

1. Know the territory. Know who the actors are, where the power is, and who is making the decisions. Keep that information current.
2. Be thoroughly grounded and familiar with legislative processes, particularly the appropriations process.
3. Maintain effective contact with legislative and agency staff.
4. Develop an effective monitoring and response mechanism.
5. Know who and what your resources are, and how and when to use them.
6. Be clear and concise in your request for assistance from officials. Learn to be patient. Results sometimes come slowly.
7. Know your competition and colleagues in the lobbying business. Know how and when to work with them on mutual problems.
8. Demonstrate an understanding of and appreciation for current economic constraints on public financing.
9. Develop an effective constituent relations program that builds public support for your group and provides constituent support for legislators sympathetic to your interest.
10. Know how and when to say thanks. There are an infinite number of ways to do this. Do not forget to do it.

Source: Remarks by Richard L. Kennedy, University of Michigan.

---

ager's role. How well the manager sets an example as a role model and how well the manager conveys his or her expectations for professionalism to the nurse greatly influences personal professionalism. Finally, the institutional milieu influences the practice of professionalism through the development of a climate conducive to autonomy, decision making, and accountability by the professionals (nurses) who are employed.

Bill patients for nursing services
separate from room charges and physician services

Most individuals working in an occupation generally referred to as a profession are reimbursed for their efforts on some sort of fee-for-service basis. At any rate, the compensation for their services is somewhat dependent on both the effort expended and their expertise and experience. This is not usually true with nursing services. Compensation by the patient for nursing services is usually hidden in some way in a daily room charge. Such a scheme causes a tremendous imbalance between the services rendered and the services paid. Someone in the hospital for a minor procedure may have the same daily charge as someone hospitalized for a more extensive procedure and needing far more care, on a relative scale.

If third-party payers would agree to reimbursement procedures based on levels of nursing care, documented by a patient classification system and posted in patient charges separate from room charges, then the costs of health care could be more equitably divided among consumers.

- Patients, upon seeing a specific charge for nursing services, might cease looking on nurses as glorified handmaidens who are "there" just like the furniture, and begin to look at them as separately compensated professionals akin to doctors, anesthetists, and so on.
- Nurses would look on *themselves* as professionals with an easily identifiable behavioral and monetary contribution to hospital operations through their services.

It must be admitted that this suggestion has an *attitudinal* impact as well. The theme permeating this book has been that organizational metamorphoses occur through changed attitudes.

Broaden orientation

Somehow, it has always been fun to send the newcomer out for an "otis elevator" or "left-handed monkey wrench." The chagrin the newcomer felt was also the first feeling of acceptance. Being new, having everything be strange is exciting; and good-natured ribbing about getting lost or taking longer is part of it.

Orientation is designed by organizations to keep this element of excitement and good-naturedness, to facilitate adaptation, and to minimize embarrassment, frustration, and inefficiency, to encourage and develop new friendships and collegiality. Nurses are oriented, aides and orderlies are oriented, dietary workers and maintenance workers are oriented. Are doctors? Are social workers? Would it not create a kinship and develop useful communication patterns to be in the same orientation group? It would also teach these valued professionals some of the nitty-gritty that would make their adaptation and job easier.

Build a better facility

The link between goodness of physical design of a hospital and the quality of care and satisfaction of the work force is tenuous at best. Yet few would argue that given the same personnel in two different physical settings, the personnel working in the newer, better equipped, and superior-designed facility would have the greater chance of giving high-quality care and receiving job satisfaction.

There are well-defined standards for the structural aspects of a hospital. There are codes or definitions concerning the load-bearing qualities of the structure, widths of halls, placement of electrical outlets, plumbing, and so on. Yet, even a structure conforming to existing codes can be unsuited for good care. Nurses who stand at their station at a hall corner and look at their area of cognizance stretching seemingly infinitely in two directions know that the physical layout is not good.

Based on their experience, nurses can give excellent input toward the design of a hospital (especially patient care areas) conducive to the best medical care. It is believed that few designers of hospitals solicit input from the major caregivers, the nurses, before finalizing a hospital's design.

There are other parts of the nuts and bolts of hospital design that can have a positive or negative effect on the mental attitude of nurses. Included among these are the following:

- The provision of a break room where the nurses can associate and socialize with each other away from the hubbub of their work. Not only does this help immensely in building an esprit de corps, but it is also excellent from the standpoint of shared experience, which can be read "education." (There might also be included a screaming room.)
- Conference rooms are needed where the nurses can be out of the work traffic pattern and have a chance to conduct meaningful meetings without interruption. These are also needed for hospitals that affiliate with collegiate and university nursing schools for student-instructor conferences.
- An adjunct to the above would be education rooms where ongoing educational sessions can be conducted without continuous work interruptions. An interrupted train of thought is difficult to get on track again.
- Offices for head nurses and patient care coordinators are necessary to ensure privacy for counseling sessions, evaluations, and supervisory and planning work.

Change your attitude

Expect no turnover. Express and exaggerate your disappointment when a nurse leaves. Be vocal about admitting failure when there are nurse exits. Investigate where things went wrong. Commit yourself to reducing turnover by one half. Enlist the total department in the campaign: "Turnover is unacceptable!"

It is not the intent of this innovation to elicit guilt all around when a nurse changes jobs. It is, however, the intent to say that *when you expect and accept turnover, it will stay at the current rate.* Nurses who are experiencing dissatisfaction will be more likely to discuss the problem in an organization that is antiturnover. This discussion is infinitely preferable to quietly slipping away; it allows the organization to change and to assess itself; and it encourages nurses to identify clearly their goals, aspirations, and discontent.

Computerize

For an industry in its infancy as late as the 1950s, digital computers have shown astounding progress. At this point, the application of computers in hospitals is limited only by the imagination of the people involved and the bankroll of the institution. As early as 1970, there were hospitals that were completely computerized from the entry of the patient (complete with the patient giving his or her own history at a computer terminal) through nurses' notes, which were computerized rather than written to a demand bill as the patient walked out of the hospital.

Discussion of the entire gamut of computer applications is beyond the scope of this book. A brief overview, however, indicates that computer usage in hospitals can be grossly divided into four areas:
- Administrative aids: patient admissions, discharge, transfer, status, census, billing, accounting
- Hospital applications: cost accounting, personnel, payroll, inventory
- Scientific management aids: use of operations research techniques in areas such as menu planning and forecasting
- Hospital results from systems: automated clinical lab results sent directly to the central computer unit and to the patient's record; automated interpretation of results such as ECGs and x-ray films.

All of the above are feasible and are being done; further, they are becoming more affordable and cost effective. One key point that should be emphasized from the beginning through to the final implementation of any computer aid is the continuing necessity of input from the planned *users* of the system. Without such input, the system has two strikes against it from the beginning.

Create annual contracts

Starting anew tends to generate optimism; fresh beginnings allow one to do better, achieve more, avoid past mistakes. New Year's resolutions, renewal of marriage vows, reaffirmations of faith allow us to begin afresh in a personal way.

Typically, we undertake professional renewal with a new job, either in a different organization or with a change in position. Entering into a new professional commitment causes one to assess and reassess self, make career choices, bargain with the hiring institution (or placement person).

Although familiarity does not always breed contempt, it does abet inactivity, laxity, and weariness. It is easy to slide along being neither stimulated nor stimulating, unaware of either pride or discouragement in the work situation. These benign feelings of usualness make one an easy target for turnover, willing prey to trying a new place for the $50 bounty or free stethoscope.

Hospitals that value retention of nurses, and thus stability in the nursing department, might do well to renegotiate with each nurse annually, combining the performance appraisal with an organization-departmental evaluation. Questions to examine might include the following:

- How are we doing about keeping our promises?
- What do you want to try next year? And how can the organization facilitate your efforts?
- Where should or could we improve? How?

The interview could end with a mutual agreement, a contract that indicates each party's goals and promises for the coming year.

Develop administrative skills

Although in recent years health care leaders have begun to recognize the need for administrative-managerial skill development, active and comprehensive planning, coordination, and efforts have been spotty. During the last two decades there has been a marked increase in the sophistication required to fill these jobs. Training and development programs are imperative. Hospitalwide efforts should be implemented. They must begin with deciding "Who should be included?" Not to be overlooked in this consideration are physicians (e.g., chiefs of staff), facility administrators, administrative board members, department heads, and nurse managers. A second question is "What skills do we need to develop?" Finally, "Who shall help us and how shall we be trained, how shall we develop?" The skill development effort in an organizational setting must from the outset include all those who may participate or who will be affected by such an effort. Two important content considerations are managerial processes (such as communication, decision making, team building, planning, modeling, and role clarification) and hospital-specific administrative information and education. As previously stated in this book, such joint activities have compounded positive effects on organization operations, norms, expectations, procedures, and values as they become clarified and often modified to meet the increased competencies of the leadership of the facility. High-quality, knowledgeable administration will lead to increased retention of professional nurses.

Exercise *professional* power

Perhaps nothing is as divisive in organizations as power: claims of power, misuse of power, and fear of power. Every person is a source of power. In a negative sense, except for infants, everyone is bigger than, stronger than, more educated than, more street-wise than, is more knowledgeable than someone else. It is, however, competitive power that prevents true teamwork. If each person is busy establishing and maintaining his or her sphere of power, others are seen as competitors and not as potential collaborators.

In a positive sense, each person has an area of expert power, a contingent of referent power. Some persons have legitimate, hierarchical power. Envisioning self and others as energy sources, as knowledge resources, builds self-concept and respect for self and others, and frees one to explore, initiate, and act.

Health care professionals share a huge responsibility, that of providing excellent health care, defining a viable health care system in a critical environment, and developing, supporting, and utilizing research efforts while encouraging and facilitating health care staff development. The task is too big for one person, one discipline; it is an undertaking that can utilize the power of all health care participants. Optimum divisions of labor and applications of all resources are possible when open discussion, mutual respect, common goals, and multidisciplinary planning are actualized.

Focus on health and hope too

Illness is a pervasive force that permeates the very core of human existence and organizational atmosphere. Traditionally, hospitals have concerned themselves with illness—treating it, researching it, fighting it. But illness is draining. The stress of curing, of healing, is itself burdensome. The stress of coping with failures, losses, disfigurement, paralysis, and death can at times be unbearable. These realities of remedial health care efforts impact heavily on the relationships of the caregivers. In fact, it is this phenomenon that greatly affects the morale of a work group. What can be done? Health care facilities must explore and carefully consider what activities and programs they can undertake that focus on prevention, promotion, and health. Structural changes should be looked at (e.g., organizationally, departmentally, or both) and efforts undertaken to bring nurses and physicians together. Each should have the opportunity to work with others under conditions of hope and innovation and normalness. Preventive and promotive medical care offer uncharted benefits for the organization, the health care professionals, the community, and society in general. The key, however, is to assure that such endeavors are integrated into the organization's operations and activities; sidelines or special units may merely polarize the facility unless, of course, careful attention is paid to rotating staff. Whatever the method, hospitals need to recognize health and healthy perspective as a part of their missions.

Institute corporate renewal programs

The concept of renewal is future oriented. Corporate renewal is based on preventive, promotive, and healthy perspectives. There are three types of renewal efforts. One consists of ongoing activities, methodologies, and structures that are built into the organization's normal work structure. Reference to these types of interventions has been made throughout this book. Activities include job rotation and enrichment, coaching, management counseling, special projects, joint goal setting, assessment committees. A second major type of renewal program is the annual off-site 3- to 5-day workshop. Its purpose is to renew (efforts, commitments, relationships, dreams), to refill (the organization and the person), and to make concrete inroads into *becoming better*—as an organization and as a professional person. Four Ps characterize such programs: promotive, preventive, participative, and productive. Such programs are usually designed by consultants in conjunction with organization representatives; activities usually include conference and case study methods, group discussions, personal time, planning, business games, and some new learning. Guidelines for preparing such programs and for participant involvement depend on the size of the system, the state of the organization, and the needs of the facility or attending group. A third type of corporate renewal program is called personal mini-retreats: these are for individuals and they usually take place when the person feels the need to look at his or her goals, to assess, to explore personal missions, to consider his or her frustrations, and to recognize limitations. Mini-retreats are legitimate renewal activities.

Corporate renewal programs encourage corporate and individual maturity, interdependence, broad-based rewards, and opportunities for self-actualization. Such goals are commensurate with the avowed objectives of hospitals and their employees.

Join the board

The composition of hospital boards has undergone restructuring and reorganization in the past decade. Attention has been given to the appointment of providers of health care as board members. The trend began slowly as one physician was appointed to the board, progressing to the point that on some boards, three fourths of the membership are physicians. As this pattern became firmly established, high-ranking hospital administrative staff (CEOs, administrators, directors of nursing) also began to be appointed to boards. Now at least one hospital in the United States (in Oregon) has a staff nurse appointed to the board.

This acknowledgment that contributions can be made to hospital governance by nurses, who comprise 50% to 70% of hospital employees, is timely and reflects a positive commitment toward correction of past impedances in recognizing the value of nursing input into the structure, policies, and procedures of the institution. This change will assist in the recruitment and retention of nursing staff and will impact positively on the delivery of quality nursing care.

It is highly desirable and recommended that the head of the nursing division or other nursing representative be appointed to the board of trustees/ directors of hospitals. Direct involvement of nursing in the decision-making process of the hospital, including membership on governing boards, is essential in order to counterbalance the traditional management view that solutions to nursing problems can be solely economic.

Learn together

Learning, grasping a new concept, drawing meaning and application from theory, recognizing in reality something from texts is a marvelous, humbling, exhilarating experience. *Sharing this experience creates bonds that last a lifetime.* Seeing things from opposite perspectives, arguing them out, disagreeing, agreeing, discussing, sharing thoughts, feelings, and perspectives are the foundations of collegiality.

There has been much written and observed about the "fraternity of doctors" and the "sisterhood of nurses"; there is an absence of the fellowship of health caregivers. Doctors tend to be educated with doctors, nurses with nurses, each in isolation from the other. Although it has been tried successfully, it is still an innovation to teach student nurses and medical students together, to have nurses teach doctors and doctors teach nurses. It is possible for hospitals to expand on this theme and build peer relating through assigning multidisciplinary teams to investigate patient complaints, accidents, errors; to research community relations; to conduct quality-assurance reviews.

It is important that all health care professions take an active role in eliminating the distance, distrust, and disregard that are rampant. It is a novel approach that caregivers come together not as competing, suspicious strangers but as teaching and learning teammates.

Let nursing be primary

Primary nursing is one way to approach the redesign of nursing care delivery systems. It shifts from a task-oriented to a process-oriented, patient-centered system, lending itself extremely well to the tenets of autonomy, authority, and accountability.

Primary nursing is an evolution from the original type of nursing care in which nurses did everything for a specific group of patients; in other words, functional assignment. The next sequence in the structure of nursing care delivery was the team approach. This fragmented patient care by assigning tasks to team members, with each nurse performing only portions of a patient's care (e.g., medications, IVs, treatments), and led to the impersonalization of patient care by making it task oriented. Primary nursing, once again, is recognized as far more rewarding.

Primary nursing is also conducive to nursing practice in collaboration with physicians and other health care professionals. In primary nursing settings nurses have developed an increased respect for the complexities of the medical management of the patient, and the physicians have come to appreciate and value the priorities of nursing care.

Primary nursing in the purest sense implies 24-hour responsibility by a designated nurse for patient care delivered to a specified group of patients. This has been adapted in a number of ways and renamed *total patient care* in some institutions. Regardless of the adaptation or name of this mode of patient care delivery, the patient knows who is responsible and accountable for the outcome of his or her care, whether for 8 hours or 24 hours, and the nurse has the authority and responsibility for a specified group of patients.

Although there are nursing and hospital administration critics of primary nursing, whether for lack of qualified staff or for economic reasons, it is still the best nursing care approach to be developed to date, which provides increased satisfaction for both nurses and patients.

Match educational and work worlds

Although this text addresses, identifies, and elaborates on many of the shortcomings of health care, nursing remains a noble profession. Thousands of professional nurses find job satisfaction, personal and professional fulfillment in practicing this profession. Although it is academically sound for nurse educators to admonish students about striving for idealistic practice and to teach under laboratory conditions, the dichotomy between education and practice is damaging to the profession. Most professions have healthy disagreement between the "ivory tower" occupants and the "real world" professionals. The relationship is healthy in its mutual stimulation. The nursing profession would gain if each side acknowledged and credited the other; thus nurses would be encouraged in their right to bring more idealism to the work setting and to identify real issues in the educational arena. Some methods of accomplishing this are listed here:

1. Have practicing nurses (directors of nursing, head nurses, staff nurses) serve as advisors to curriculum committees in schools of nursing.
2. Have head nurses work with clinical instructors to make assignments for students.
3. Stop tolerating one another and confront each other!
4. Schedule students for realistic work hours and assignments toward the end of training.
5. Have nurse educators serve as advisors to (or members of) quality-assurance, procedure, staffing committees.
6. Join together to halt the severe culture shock that prompts so many to exit from the profession.

Nurses: Involve yourselves in the community

Nurses must become involved in community affairs. Although they have in recent years been more visible as hospitals and other agencies have taken on home-based care and preventive teaching activities, both of these are limited to nurses' roles as caregivers. Nursing must expand its orientation, and one way is through social action. It is this social action phenomenon that is highly representative in the maturation process of a profession. Nursing must mature as a profession, therefore nurses must undertake more visible and numerous social action endeavors. Businesses support and encourage their employees to become involved in the community. Hospitals and other health care facilities must do the same. Hospitals must recognize the total person, and thus they must value and broaden the spectrum of involvement of nurses. Nurses have much to offer such volunteer groups as United Way, Junior Achievement, health fairs; such political activities as voter registration drives, information forums, and fund raising; additionally, nurses must recognize their contributions as parents, as churchgoers, as neighborhood representatives. The more professionally nurses are encouraged and allowed to behave—and the more professional they become through their own actions—the more likely nurses will stay, will retain their allegiance with the organization with which they identify and with which the community identifies them. Contributing to the community, promoting the profession, providing visibility for the health care facility, and recognizing the fullness of human life are all benefits and outcomes of this innovation.

Nurses: Take your rightful place in administration

The nursing profession is 98% female; the profession of nursing is a nurturing one. Neither of these is a negative leadership quality. However, nurturing women have been exploited, set up, and taken advantage of in health care.

"Typically, nursing control is perceived at the level of patient care units but not at the organizational level. Nursing was seen as a frequent victim of encroachment by others."[9] "Nurses are not consulted frequently enough by the medical staff about matters on which nurses could give good advice."[2] "The female can win individual plays but the game itself must be won by the male. The socialization of a little girl dictates that she must learn how to lose. She is supposed to acquiesce and please whomever is master."[3]

Historic and socialized expectations and behaviors make it difficult for nursing leaders to assert themselves. Nevertheless, more nurses are appearing on boards of directors and on administrative committees, and are exerting their influence, defending their beliefs, and relying on their expert power. Assertive (not aggressive or passive-aggressive) nurse leaders are a welcome, needed, and significant innovation. They are pioneers.

Perform organizational assessments (the Phoenix process)

Organizational development (OD) is described and put into operation in Chapter 8. Within such endeavors is the process of regular and planned organizational assessments. Usually these assessments occur annually and encourage broad-based participation. In hospitals this includes board of directors, physician, nurse, community member, patient, administrator, and departmental representative. Examples of assessment methods include attitude surveys, review of "hard data" such as turnover rates or other specific information, and managerial styles questionnaires. The types of assessments should be determined according to a 5-year assessment master plan in combination with the group(s) or concern (e.g., retention) targeted for more in-depth focus. Once data are collected and analyzed, action steps are determined and defined that have as their major purpose the enhancement of organizational and personal efficiency and effectiveness. Although action steps are based on the specific needs gleaned from the survey process, some general categories include training, communications, career counseling, productivity, employee recognition, team building, and task forces. The entire Phoenix process (so named by us after the ongoing organizational assessment effort of the city of Phoenix, Arizona) is a learning experience that improves managerial abilities of participants/team members. It further enhances personal development and organizational well-being. Readers are encouraged to review the section on OD in Chapter 8 for concrete "how to's" in implementing such diagnostic procedures. Most importantly, having a sense of "where we are now," with data to support that sense, can provide the much-needed guidelines for how organizations can change for the sake of improvement.

Program for retirement

At this time, relatively few nurses actually "retire" from nursing in the sense of working productively at nursing as a career until the age of retirement mandated in the institution's personnel policies. Perhaps more often, nurses "retire" from burnout or frustration, or they simply enter a more lucrative field.

Suppose conditions change as suggested within this book. Suppose most nurses begin to work actively in the field of nursing until they are ready to actually retire from the profession. What then? Nursing is a very stressful profession, but it is also a profession where one has a sense of being needed, day after day. If this impetus for living—the feeling of being needed—is removed suddenly, it may have a tremendously deleterious effect on the health and well-being, both physical and mental, of the retiree. An indication might be taken from the history of military retirees in this country. When a person who has been in a regimented, stressful, usually closely controlled situation all his or her adult life is suddenly cut loose of responsibilities while still at a productive age, she or he often becomes lost or even dies quickly. One tack taken by the military to soften the blow of retirement has been to have pre-retirement planning and counseling available for those soon to retire.

This type of system can also be used with nurse retirees. At some predetermined time before actual retirement, planning sessions should be set up. Some possible ways to help a nurse prepare for retirement are as follows:

- Gradually cut down on the hours worked from full-time to quarter-time.
- Nurses at or closely approaching retirement age can fill in gaps in coverage.
- Some retiring nurses can be encouraged to act as mentors for newly graduated nurses, easing their transition by making available their clinical expertise as well as their knowledge of hospital operations and procedures.
- Retired nurses can be well utilized in a public relations capacity for speaking engagements, health fairs, and so on.

Provide day (and night) care

The concept of hospitals providing day-care centers for employees' children is not a new one. For many years, there has been an occasional hospital in a certain geographic location that has constructed, annexed, or found a suitable area within the institution for the provision of child care services for the children of hospital employees, 24 hours a day. Some institutions with day-care centers have even provided isolated areas to take care of employee's children who were ill, segregating them from well children. This was particularly attractive to nurses who had to work evening or night shifts. However, because of the expense involved in establishing and operating day-care centers, along with the liability involved for the hospital, this service has never been widespread.

The hospital-owned and -operated day-care center is an ideal structure particularly if it is set up for 24-hour service. However, this is not always possible or even feasible for a hospital. In these cases there are several viable alternatives. One is a contract with a nearby day-care center for which the child care expenses of employees' children are either totally or partially reimbursed by the hospital. Another variation of this is to allow employees to choose any licensed day-care center for their children and submit their expenses to the hospital for partial or full reimbursement. This type of repayment can be classified as nontaxable income for the employee and provide a real benefit in savings.

Day-care benefits are a source of employee gain that should be made available for all employees, and eligibility should not be restricted to only full-time or only female employees. Also, reimbursement should be available not only for employees who need child care while they work but also for employees who work the night shift and who must have day care for children while they sleep.

Ratio output to input

The efficiency of any activity can be measured by ratioing output to input. Within a production environment, when output diminishes, input can also be reduced to keep the ratio within an acceptable range. This may be accomplished by shutting down an assembly line, closing out a shift of workers, or other alternative means.

The same types of general techniques are also valid in a health care environment. This, of course, would be partially dependent on the initial physical design of a hospital. In general, people do not like to be in a hospital over the weekend. It should be possible to shut down selected units if they are not needed. Such a step requires the coordination of several efforts.

- The hospital design must be such as to make it cost effective (as well as possible) to shut down a unit. Doors could be locked and air-conditioning ducts could be shut off. Lighting could be cut. Nursing stations could be located in such a manner as to allow the efficient shutdown of a unit.
- The part of the admissions process having to do with the assignment of rooms must be apprised of what is going on and must cooperate with the effort.

Another possibility of enhancing efficiency is in the area of setting up individual cost centers and having nurses' monetary rewards at least partially based on the operational efficiency of the unit. Safeguards must be built into such schemes to ensure that nurses balance the efficiency of the unit against the quality of care so that scrimping will not be a temptation. Operating on such a cost center basis is an excellent ground for training nurses in all the aspects of financial administration for movement upward in the hierarchy.

Redraw the organization chart

One continual source of frustration to a nurse is in the organizational structure and the attendant reporting structure. Nurses are caregivers, yet their reporting structure is through the administrative side of the organization. In the traditional structure, the director of nursing reports to the administrator. As discussed in Chapter 6, a large part of a nurse's activities involves a certain amount of managing and administration, even for a staff nurse. However, the main reason for a nurse's being in the hospital is as a caregiver.

Why not have the nurses report to the medical side of the organization? A physician, perhaps with a master's degree in hospital administration, could have a title on the order of director of patient care. Reporting to such a person would be the director of nursing and the chief of staff. Any differences arising between nurses and physicians could be arbitrated by a medically trained person with responsibility for both groups instead of having two groups, one with a medically trained and one with an administratively trained person at the head, attempt to settle a dispute. Such an organization structure would have a number of benefits:

- It would put nurses on a much more equal footing with the physicians, hierarchically, as befits their training, experience, and contributions.
- It would be ideal for the development of patient care teams. The physician remains the primary source of medical care, with input from the nurse. The assigned nurse in each team becomes *administrative* head of each team, with formally defined authority over the remaining members of the team. The team members are still under the authority of their functional heads, but are subject to the *project* authority of the administrative head of the team, the nurse. This innovation builds on the concept of matrix organization designs so relevant to hospital systems.

The arrangement described above should help considerably, both in enhancing nurses' feelings of professionalism and in ensuring maximum coordination of patient care.

Rewards—more than money

In many areas, the nursing profession and hospitals have lagged behind other industries in the provision of benefits taken for granted in other professions. Many of these benefits are unique to a primarily female profession, and some are more generally applicable. Some possible benefits to be added are listed here.

Salaries. Salary scales should be developed that are commensurate with the responsibilities of nurses as professionals and caregivers in our nation's health care institutions. These may include the following:

- Differentials for BSN, MSN educational preparation
- Differentials for National Specialty Certification
- Differentials for evening and night shifts
- Differentials for weekends
- Merit salary increases tied to performance

Educational opportunity. Time off or flexible scheduling should be available to meet class requirements for obtaining nursing degrees. Other assistance might include tuition reimbursement, full educational assistance (tuition, books, time off in conjunction with contract to hospital), and education days (1 week per year) to attend workshops and seminars.

Relocation. Many professions take for granted some help with relocation expenses. Good nurses are hard to find and may need help moving.

Parking. Nearby parking provided by the hospital is helpful. Requiring a nurse to pay a monthly parking fee from an already meager salary adds insult to injury.

Car pooling. Aid in setting up car pooling or van pooling to or from an inner-city location cuts down greatly on the hassle involved in getting to work.

Stock. Provision of a stock purchase plan in a for-profit institution gives a feeling of commitment to and ownership in the organization.

Bank of days. Holidays, vacation, and sick time, accumulated according to longevity with the institution, can be taken at any time during the year; employees also can take pay for a certain percentage of earned days in lieu of time off.

Safety benefits. A good combination of insurance, retirement, and annuities available to nurses will go far toward instilling in them a feeling that the organization cares about what happens to them. In addition, if there is a valid reason for a nurse to leave the institution, she can do so without the sinking feeling that she is going to end up "old and broke" with no retirement benefits accrued.

All employees' benefits have to be individualized depending on the organization and its ability to finance and undertake such programs. The most successful benefit packages have been developed by task forces or committees composed of employee representatives and administration.

Set goals together

The process of goal setting has clearly been recognized as the basis on which organizations and groups can determine their future and assess their progress. In recent years joint activities have gained much attention as functional togetherness has greatly influenced the quality of the product and the participants' commitment to same. This participative strategy is probably nowhere more important than in the goal-setting process—of an organization, a department, or a unit—whether the emphasis is on short- or long-range goals. Annual hospitalwide goal setting is a most imperative area to encourage participative management. The broader the representation in this process, the greater likelihood a sense of team consciousness in mission will occur. Also, because of clarity regarding the goals, day-to-day adjustments are more likely to be based on goals and outcomes (task) rather than artificial elements such as whims, status, power, or lack of understanding. Utilization of joint goal-setting methodology within various departmental groups is the key. Another joint goal-setting strategy is the utilization of ad hoc committees to meet special circumstances or to consider new programs for facility growth and development. Physicians, staff nurses, and nurse managers, as well as pharmacy, dietary, and x-ray personnel can be jointly involved in defining medical goals. In considering institutional goals, no representative employee or community group should be omitted. In generating administrative-managerial guidelines, all persons charged with managing and supervising must come together.

Staff creatively

One of the most promising employee incentives to attract nurses to hospitals in recent years was borrowed from industry after being used successfully in Japan and Europe. It is commonly called flexible scheduling or flextime. It has been the most successful of all tactics in coaxing unemployed nurses back to hospitals. Often it has been coupled with nurse refresher or reorientation programs to attract those nurses back to the work setting who have been inactive in the profession for a period of time. The adaptations of flexible scheduling are limited only to one's imagination and creative propensities. Some of the more frequently seen are listed in Chapter 5.

Support each other

Stress and burnout are two common phenomena in nursing today. "Administrators as well as nurses themselves are becoming aware that the 'giving,' so much a part of nursing care, must be balanced by a 'receiving' or 'refueling' for the nurse herself."[5] The ability to help support one another is predicated on respect, caring, and investment in one another.

The organization can facilitate staff supportiveness, or it can undermine and prevent such efforts. When staff spending time with staff is seen as derelict from duty, support will not occur. When staff lounges and coffee break rooms are used for storage, helping occurs rarely.

This "innovation" is not really new. It has been organized, legitimized, even facilitated by outside experts. However, being supportive, reaching out to co-workers, sharing one's feelings (hurts, frustrations, and exaltations) on a day-to-day basis require commitment and work.

Nurses are visible on the front line; their need for support has been noted and researched. Physicians also invest, hurt, experience frustration and despair. They can (and do) respond to support; they also need to be refilled. Reaching out, supporting, investing, confronting, comforting, and being authentic with co-workers (nurse to nurse, nurse to doctor, aide to nurse) can do nothing but strengthen both quality of patient care and self-esteem/self-actualization of health caregivers.

Take collegiality seriously

Collegiality is a vague term but one of unquestionable value to organizations and people. Collegiality implies an aura of positive relationships, accepted contributions, mutual support, and sense of teamwork. It relies on organizational climate, policies, and activities, as well as on individual personal behaviors such as reaching out, listening, asking, accepting, giving, confronting, and valuing. Collegiality is hard work and requires investment by both the organization and its membership. An innovation for health care is to work toward consciously bridging gaps: between management and staff, physicians and nurses, patients and admitting or accounts receivable, X-ray department and nursing, purchasing and food services, surgery and pediatrics, director of nursing and administrator, regulating agencies and hospital leadership/legal counsel. Collegiality requires formal, stated perspectives about the organizational attitude vis-à-vis working together. Multidisciplinary collegiality is crucial to this process. Medical and administrative relationships (within and between each) must be reexamined and clarified in light of their common goals. That is the starting point: reinforcing the commonness of the mission of the organization among its human resources—nurses, physicians, accountants, receptionists, ward clerks, orderlies. A first step is to determine in crossrepresentative groups: "How do we define collegiality in this organization? How shall we define it for the future?"

Tend to your present employees

Hospitals should be as concerned for the physical and emotional health of their employees as they are for their patients. Therefore, time and attention must be given to the development of programs and systems that promote wellness. Some ideas for programs are the following:

- Stop smoking programs
- Weight control programs
- Employee health screening and counseling clinics
- Leisure-time activities (team sports, classes, trips, concerts)
- Physical fitness programs (gyms, spas, jogging tracks, tennis courts, aerobic conditioning programs)
- Stress reduction techniques
- Positive mental attitude programs
- Financial planning and counseling
- Community resource referral service

Treat culture shock properly

Yes, new graduates experience a shock when entering full-time employment. This is true of all professions. Nursing may be unique as it deals with life and death, with crippling disease, altered self-concepts, difficult choices (euthanasia, brain death, donor care). And it feels very vulnerable, very alone to be a professional, to claim to be able to deal and cope with life's very heavy issues.

Transition from student nurse to graduate nurse usually also signals transition from child to adult, from dependent to independent, from supervised to accountable, from passive to active. Every choice seems more significant, more important, more visible, more long lasting, and one is left to make choices alone. More is expected and less is given. Transition is very stressful.

Health care organizations have chosen to deal with this weighty transition with lengthy orientation programs, internships, and the like. The emphasis is on one's clinical and technical expertise. Few professions demand as much technical learning as does the profession of nursing. It seems highly possible that some personal growth, self-awareness, and personal maturation are sacrificed to that end. Yet it is these components that bring about "culture shock" and that cause some nurses to abandon the profession to fill roles less personally demanding.

The profession should examine this phenomenon.

Use pools for swimming

Supplemental agency help is often helpful, but it only temporarily assuages the institution's nursing shortage or ineffectual leadership. The nursing pool has a place in health care (e.g., home health services), but that place is *not* in an ongoing team effort, in a hospital or other health care institution. Agency help is more expensive than on-staff personnel, and less knowledgeable regarding specific patients and the specific organization.

The benefits professional nurses achieve by working through a "pool" are attainable through a number of creative options designed by the institutions. It is less costly and greatly advantageous for the organization to explore some of these alternatives.

Ongoing, significant requests for supplemental help should be a red flag to nursing administration. It indicates a patch of illness, of weakness in the nursing department, a symptom not to be overlooked or quickly labeled but seriously and thoroughly investigated.

Utilize inventory wisely

As has been stated previously, a hospital is a very labor-intensive operation. The operation, however, runs on supplies. If the supplies are not available at the appropriate place, at the proper time, in the correct amounts, it may still be possible to give a semblance of good care, but only at the expense of more time and effort (and frustration) on the part of nurses.

Good systems exist for the management of inventories and the distribution of those inventories. Although it may seem desirable in a hospital always to have excesses of all supplies, this is neither possible nor efficient. Other industries have practiced scientific management of inventories for a number of years. The application is effective in both theory and practice. Good inventory management that minimizes dollar investment while still maintaining adequate supplies can free a substantial amount of money for other purposes. Such systems are readily computerized.

In addition to the above, systems are available that can help to manage the distribution of the inventory. Suppose, for example, that a "bill of materials" is made up for the more common procedures done in hospitals. By forecasting the demand for these various procedures, the items to be used can be ordered in time to arrive, be prepackaged, and be available to be taken to wherever they are needed.

A good system of ordering supplies based on valid rationales, and of logging them in, out, and back in as needed, can go far in (1) keeping investment in unneeded supplies to a minimum and (2) keeping the frustration factor resulting from unavailable necessities at a minimum.

Work for quality

The reputation of a company for building or furnishing a quality product has a bearing on the satisfaction felt by people working there. An employee who feels compelled to defend a work place continually against allegations of poor quality does not generally make a satisfied employee. Over the long term, such feelings have an impact on personnel turnover. Because stakes in the "product" are high and the effect of poor quality is emotional, health care professionals are no exceptions to the above argument.

Hypothesize that better feelings about an institution in terms of quality of care will lead to increased commitment to retain one's employment at that institution. It should follow, then, that a good quality-assurance program that helps to ensure high-quality care influences in a positive manner a nurse's decision to stay.

There have been and will continue to be arguments about the best method to measure the quality of care, as well as whether or not it *can* be measured. Nevertheless, there are methods that give *indicators* of quality. A hospital might best address the question by using a spectrum of methods. Inside the hospital, statistical analyses may be computed on admissions to the hospital, outcome of care, and committee reports (such as the tissue committee). Other measures might be used that are based on control charting of nursing care, the patient environment, and other visible indicators. Additional information is available from interviews with departing patients or from questionnaires.

Information taken from all these sources, and *acted on,* can measurably improve the *apparent* and real quality of care at an institution.

Work *with* the union

An innovation in dealing with unions is for hospital leaders to work with these groups from a posture of cooperativeness to recognize a mutuality of purpose. Administrators must begin to ask a whole new set of questions with regard to union negotiations: "What are our common goals for the year?" "How can we support employees in the process of achieving these goals?" "How will the unions support the process?" Too often the adversary relationship between organization and union representatives has put progress on hold while each connives and manipulates, downgrades and calls names. The result is the creation of an atmosphere that undermines healthy and productive work efforts. There is nothing wrong with an organization whose sole purpose is to secure the well-being of its members, and unions do just that. Health care facilities must examine their intentions; at the core they are probably the same intentions as those of the union, particularly as they relate to achieving corporate goals. Why cannot the two groups, then, sit down to determine goals that are commensurate with each representative group's criteria? Creative problem solving can be utilized to define legitimate, knowledgeable conditions for employee and organizational well-being. At the center, the intentions of each group are compatible. Strategies and *actions* must be implemented to build on this compatibility. A first step—the first risk—can come from hospital leadership: approach union representatives and institute negotiations *before* the formal contractual period is up. Cut through traditional meetings, times, and formats. And, most importantly, eliminate "middlemen." Try cooperation. It may take many tries and years, but it can enhance this crucial relationship.

REFERENCES AND ADDITIONAL READINGS

1. Adapted from remarks by R. Kennedy, Vice-President for State Relations, University of Michigan.
2. Bates, F.L., and White, R.F.: Differential perceptions of authority in hospitals, J. Health & Soc. Behav. **2**(4):265, 1961.
3. Cleland, V.: Sex discrimination: nursing's most pervasive problem, Am. J. Nurs. **71**(8):1545, Aug. 1971.
4. Davis, C.K., Pakley, D., and Sochalski, J.A.: Leadership for expanding nursing influence on health policy, J. Nurs. Admin. **12**:20, Jan. 1982.
5. Scully, R.: Staff support groups: helping nurses to help themselves, J. Nurs. Admin. **11**(3):48, March 1981.
6. Velthouse, B., and Vogt, J.F.: Colleagial helping: am I my colleagues' keeper?, Unpublished article, 1982.
7. Vereyen, L.G.: Change through employee feedback, Train. & Develop. J. **33**(9): 40-43, Sept. 1979.
8. Vogt, J.F.: Corporate renewal, a presentation for the Milwaukee Bar Association, April 17, 1980.
9. Weisman, C.S., Alexander, C.L.S., and Morlock, L.L.: Hospital decision making: what is nursing's role? J. Nurs. Admin. **11**(9):33, Sept. 1981.

8

PLANNING FOR CHANGE AND CHANGING: ORGANIZATIONAL DEVELOPMENT

We believe retention is tied to the foundation of organizational activities and operations. This chapter explores this relationship in light of change. Change is sorely needed in regard to the retention of staff nurses; it is also appropriate to hospital management, administration, structure and design, missions, and goals. It is beyond the scope of this book to explore and define organizational change and development in depth. However, it has been the experience of the authors that "change begets change." This has been noted in the consultation activities of Vogt-Velthouse Associates.

> As we have worked with nurses and nursing management, it has been our experience that growth, crises, change, and improvements have reflected and impacted throughout the hospital environment. Nurses can and do make a difference in the total scheme of health. It is crucial that they know how much influence they have and that they are later willing to take responsibility for facilitating change as it evolves within the organization. Perhaps more importantly it is necessary to help the various hospital departments, groups, and leaders outside of nursing to be aware of the effect nursing's development will have on them.[30]

There is something very fundamental about changing to improve—especially changing that promotes the retention of nurses. It may be the issues of personal motivation, of stability, of crises, of health and health care, of human valuing human, and of *keeping* versus losing. Whatever the issue, it will reach every dimension of hospital activity. Change is inevitable.

The cost of high turnover among nurses is staggering. *The process of designing and effecting planned retention will result in far-reaching organizational growth and development.* As with any change, the process is often painful, often a struggle, fraught with highs and lows. The trade-off is not as simple as taking a pill. The fact is, the medical model is the antithesis of the kinds of planned change activities that will make a lasting dent in a hospital's high rate of turnover. Planned retention methodologies require time, personal investment, commitment, and dollars. They require a broad base of support. And they require an objective resource—usually an organizational change consultant (or group) who understands, values, and can facilitate *healthy change.* The tools, ideas, and specific concepts for improving retention lie *within* the organization; sometimes experts have inputs that are especially meaningful as well. However, it is the gathering of these ideas, selecting those that fit the particular organization, implementing strategies, and committing selves to the "whole of the process" as well as to the specifics undertaken that are imperatives. This is the *process* of planned retention, and it requires an organizational change and development expert who can stay with the organization for the life of the change. The person may be internal or external to the system, but this expert, we believe, is basic to success.

The change process alluded to above and the concept of planned retention advocated here have their roots in the principles, theory, and practice of planned change and organizational development. In effect, we are defining planned retention through these precepts. Readers are urged to strengthen their knowledge base beyond this chapter's input. One of the soundest sources for historical, current, and applied information is the Addison-Wesley Series on Organizational Development[4,22]; it is a most appropriate addition to the library of any organization undergoing such activities. Since the early 1970s a whole new field of study has emerged in business school curriculums across the country: organizational behavior. Organizational development (OD) and change have spawned this new area of inquiry and learning in a rather short time span (about 35 years), and it is within this new area of scientific and philosophical examination that one will find most OD efforts. For those readers who do not have a working knowledge of organizational behavior, we encourage you to seek out such knowledge actively. Course work alone is not going to be sufficient for the issues at hand. For that reason, we urge that persons wanting true help in these areas demand learning that is called experiential. *Experiential learning* is synonymous with OD and planned change constructs. It is basic to those goals. When asking about courses, workshops, seminars, and consultation activities, be sure to qualify the offerings by assuring that they are built on the principles of experiential education and are staffed by persons trained in experiential education design, methodologies, values, and ethics. (See box on p. 236 entitled, What is "Experiential Education?")

The purpose of this book is to go beyond the simplistic and narrow solutions being proffered to solve the problems of nursing turnover. It is our perspective that effective retention strategies are those that are (1) planned, (2) specific to the needs and circumstances of the facility, (3) constantly assessed and updated, and (4) based on the principles of human resource management, (5) while focusing on opportunities and innovations within the entire organization. A common thread that runs through this perspective is the belief that professional people want to grow, want to contribute, and want to be valued. The health care organization that fosters and encourages these human conditions will *retain* productive, self-fulfilled nurse professionals.

Issues of retention are deeply imbedded within the operations of the organization. Therefore, rather than merely focusing on change as it relates to retention, this chapter focuses on the broader picture: organizational change. Issues related specifically to retention are dealt with and examined within their proper perspective and place in the organizational change process. The major topics of this chapter are the process of change, phases of organizational development (OD), the people in OD, and the impact of change.

This chapter represents a sound basis for starting; and starting is the essence of planned retention. It offers theoretical, concrete, and practical dis-

WHAT IS EXPERIENTIAL EDUCATION?

DEFINITION

Experiential education is a cyclical process. After immediate concrete experiences learners observe and reflect on their activities; their observations are brought together to form a "theory" from which new implications for their behavior are generated; these implications then serve as guides for learners as they practice new learning experiences.

ALSO CALLED LABORATORY EDUCATION

In laboratory learning, learners participate in and reflect on many kinds of activities; their principal concern is their own behavior—their "selves." The learning emphasis is on the "here-and-now" behaviors of participants.

OUTCOMES

Learners tend to "learn" the following from experiential education environments:
• Expanded consciousness of their world
• Recognition of choice in life's experiences
• A spirit of inquiry—a willingness to ask
• Authenticity, that is, realness in interpersonal relations
• A collaborative perception of authority relationships

EXPERIENTIAL EDUCATION FACILITATOR DESIGN SKILLS

The role of facilitators is multifaceted. One of their key roles is to design laboratory learning. Five skills are of primary importance in order for effective experiential education to occur:
1. Ability to identify specific and explicit learning goals of the activity(s)
2. Sensitivity to and anticipation of participant responses and receptivity to the design
3. Ability to sequence learning activities
4. Ability to collaborate meaningfully and noncompetitively with other facilitators
5. Ability to modify and redirect the design while events are in progress

EXPERIENTIAL EDUCATION LEARNING COMPONENTS

There are five major components or activity types used in experiential education:
1. Intensive small groups
2. Structured learning experiences
3. Lecturettes/handouts (theory input)
4. Self-time
5. Back-home applications

AS DISTINGUISHED FROM TRADITIONAL EDUCATION

Traditional education focuses on processes meant to help plastic learners acquire the skills and information necessary to negotiate a fixed cultural environment.

Experiential education sees learning as a transaction between a fluid and unfixed learner and environment; each therefore undergoes change.

cussions regarding both *what* to do and *how* to do it. It is the nature and strength of this what/how relationship that will determine the success of the organizational development effort and its impact on retention.

THE PROCESS OF CHANGE

The concept of organizational change is not new; however, the current focuses regarding this concept are. Traditionally, it has been recognized that organizations have experienced pressure to change from three sources: (1) technical innovation, (2) competition and the struggle for survival (usually economic), and (3) participants' increasing requests for freedom and self-direction within organizational settings. In recent years there has been an ever-increasing social tendency on the part of individuals to transform their dependence on organizations into beneficial interdependence between personal worth and organizational affluence. Any of the above three pressures for change—technical, economic, and social—can determine the change targets and the change strategy. Each is also associated with a certain concept of organization. For example, the *technical* concept translates into an organization consisting of a collection of specialized tasks and procedures that are coordinated for the purpose of making a product or delivering a service. The usual method of change is to redesign the work-flow patterns and educate accordingly. This method of change usually has limited success, does not affect attitudes, and utilizes legitimate authority. The *survival* concept of organization usually centers on the structure of authority and formalized power through position—the main purpose of organization being to control behavior for the sake of predictability and unity. Change here usually occurs through forced compliance. Such change involves observable acts, prompts negative reactions, and does not include reeducation. The *social* concept perceives the organization as a system of dynamically interdependent people who are involved in the process of decision making, communicating, norm setting, rewarding, and punishing. The major organizational purpose is collaborating and adapting to the environment. Change methods here include shared decision making and open dialogue about goals, strategies, norms, and needs satisfaction. These methods work when employees participate in decision making in proportion to their capabilities, when they see their input utilized, and when they are able to make decisions skillfully and comfortably. Unfortunately, each of these change strategies vis-à-vis simplistic organizational definitions is no longer viable in and of itself. Rational, reeducative, or power-coercive changes are insufficient given the conditions of today's work world.

"We are living in a world that calls for a certain continuous alert apprehensiveness. . . . This is one of the most exciting things about our present decade—that the community will not tolerate things that would have been

TABLE 8-1
Trends in the movement from disappearing bureaucracy
to emerging adhocracy*

Disappearing bureaucracy	Emerging adhocracy
OLD CULTURE	**NEW CULTURE**
A system characterized by more permanence, hierarchy, and division of labor	Fast-moving, information-rich, kinetic organization of the future
Traditionally, workers labored in sharply defined slots or roles with narrow specializations	Modern systems with transient units, mobile personnel, and continuous reorganization
Workers operated within a chain of command from the top down	Workers' roles more hazy and temporary in a setting where talents and disciplines converge to accomplish task
Somewhat intractable structures and departments	Fluid, participative arrangements with changing organizational roles, relationships, and structures
Slow to change, usually as a result of external influences	
Somewhat static in operations	Characterized by disposable divisions, task forces, project teams, and ad hoc units
Primarily concerned about self-interests of organization	Sense of corporate social responsibility
Functions well in stable society where problems are routine and predictable, environment is competitive and undifferentiated	Dynamic, self-renewing, continuously adapting
	Functions best in a super-industrial society of cyberculture characterized by accelerating change
Vertical power concentration among a few at top levels who make all important decisions for lower echelons	Horizontal disbursement of power with a shift of decisions sideways and to lower levels of responsibility
Organizational communication is vertical, slow, and delay is normal	More sharing of decision making with workers and consumers, and wider input
Simple problem-solving mechanisms for routine issues and low speed decisions	Organizational communications circular or lateral with fast information flow and computerized systems; delay costly
Staff/line arrangements between support and operative units	Complex problem solving for meeting increasingly nonroutine, novel, and unexpected problems requiring high speed decisions
Required mass of moderately educated workers for routine performance	Team approach with convergence of specializations
Emphasis on efficiency, profitability, plant/equipment, maintenance, and capital expansion	Requires fewer knowledge workers and technicians
	Emphasis on people and human resource development
OLD ORGANIZATION MAN	**NEW ASSOCIATION PERSON**
Frequently a white male who employs his energies and skills for the good of the organization to whom he is loyal and committed	Varied competent people, including many women and minorities, who employ their energies and skills for self-actualization, often in temporary groupings
Considers executives and managers the "brains," while workers are the "hands"	Mobile, self-motivated persons who take economic security for granted, and seek personal and professional development
Labors within a hierarchical pyramid in which rank and role are clearly defined	

*From Harris, P.R.: Innovating with high achievers in HRD, p. 46.

TABLE 8-1—cont'd
Trends in the movement from disappearing bureaucracy
to emerging adhocracy

Disappearing bureaucracy	Emerging adhocracy
Looks to the corporation or agency for approval and recognition, reward and punishment	See executives and managers as coordinators/consultants of mixed, temporary work teams
Conditioned somewhat to subservience and paid to conform; discouraged from displaying creativity or deviancy	Operate in complex setting, within a matrix requiring flexibility and functional skills
Concerned about economic security and status in the organization, subordinating individuality for the good of the organization	Often creative deviants who look within self and profession for approval and fulfillment
	Knowledgeable workers who respect only the authority of competence
Joins in corporate emphasis on competition, success, and achieving quantity production	Skilled in human relations and group dynamics so as to be capable of quick, intense work relationships on a temporary team, and then disengaging for another challenging assignment
Usually a narrow specialist with limited education who fears change, and advocates the status quo	
By his past orientation, is ripe for future shock	Agents of change who find transience liberating and emphasize cooperation and quality production or service
The exceptional among his type were the free-swinging entrepreneurs who built vast enterprises, fiercely defining rugged individualism and independence, in the spirit of western pioneers	Individuals who create and plan their future, envisioning change as a challenge for new learning
	These superindustrial persons are often entrepreneurial groups, sometimes within large, complex systems in which interdependence is the norm
	Unafraid to enter into new fields, and even to pioneer the universe

tolerated . . . in another age." With these words Margaret Mead[19] has identified two of the most disquieting conditions visible in today's organizations: the need to be aware of new circumstances and the realization that people have grown in behalf of themselves. As a result, organizational models and managerial styles of the century thus far are no longer as appropriate or effective. Philip Harris[12] has characterized the current adjustments in organizational life as movement from "disappearing bureaucracy" to "emerging adhocracy," from classical-authoritarian to participative-matrix. Table 8-1 summarizes the trends that have become a part of this broadly based transition. It is these conditions that made the dearth of knowledge about change so apparent and so painful to organizations and persons needing to change. It is this movement that eventually spawned planned change. It is fortunate that work had begun in the 1940s that served as the basis for and met the needs being felt regarding change.

Planned change

By the late 1950s, this work emerged into the concepts of planned change. It is this construct and its practical applications and implications that have greatly altered the chances for success and the quality of success in to-day's organizations. Bennis et al.[5] define planned change as a "conscious, deliberate, and collaborative effort to improve the operations of a system through the utilization of scientific knowledge." In their pioneering work, *The Planning of Change*, they identified five major areas basic to planned change: its creation, implementation, evaluation, and maintenance; the fifth area focuses on resistance to change. Some of the most significant contributions made by planned change practitioners and thinkers are described here:

- The change process
- Stages of change
- Principles of change
- Resistance to change
- Acceptance of change
- Readiness
- The change agent and ethics

The change process

The father of group dynamics, planned change, and organizational development is Kurt Lewin.[14] His research and theory building of the late 1930s and the 1940s created the most firm foundation in the shortest amount of time for any significant body of knowledge with applied activities in academic history. The present volume has literally taken the opportunity to "return to the basics" by referring to the extensive contributions of Kurt Lewin (see Chapters 3 and 4 on team building and motivation). It is Lewin's conceptualization of change that is of primary importance to us here. Lewin conceived of a system (organization, person, group) as "frozen." In order to change, he said, the system must *"unfreeze,"* then *"change,"* and then *"refreeze."* To help the reader get a vivid understanding of these elements, we suggest that you picture in your mind a river frozen solid through the cold winter months of the North. Watch that river as a warming trend begins: it gradually melts and thaws (decreasing the thickness of the ice and shrinking away from its banks), until ice floes are rapidly rushing downstream (the river often overflowing and tearing out debris as it moves). The river is unfreezing. Change occurs: the shapes of the banks, the floor of the riverbed, its source and mouth may be altered. Once the change has occurred, the river must refreeze; perhaps the water level goes down and allows for a solid, normal flow of water (as in the warm summer months), or perhaps it is the gradual freezing of a new winter— and the process continues.

In conceiving change in this manner, Lewin[14] and his colleagues (Zander,[33] Cartwright, Lippitt,[15,16] and others) recognized that the work that lay ahead consisted of identifying and designing means to facilitate this movement, in defining various steps in the process, in recommending organizational activities, in considering and involving human emotions and feelings. But just as the unfreezing–change–refreezing process of the river is *natural,* so they believed change must spring from the system itself; it must in some way fit the conditions of the system. It is through a realization that change is normal and natural that Lewin and colleagues began to explore the role of change agent as helper and expert in the change *process,* not as the recommender of change. (More about the change agent can be found on pp. 273-280 of this chapter.) Change is as inevitable as the seasons. Lewin conceived of the role of change agents as that of helping people and organizations deal effectively with this fact of existence.

Stages of change

The concept of the unfreezing–changing–refreezing process of change led to the recognition that there were steps that could be followed to prompt change appropriate to the system. Early work carried out at the University of Michigan's Center for Research on Utilization of Scientific Knowledge recommended four steps to improve change efforts:

1. Systematic diagnosis of the system (structure, person, organization) to be changed
2. Diagnosis of the possibilities and limitations for change
3. Development of an action plan for initiating and maintaining the change
4. Continuous evaluation and replanning as the change effort progresses

Perhaps the single most significant contribution made by early thinkers has to do with data gathering and diagnosis. Planned change rests on the firm conviction that there is a need for change, and there are demonstrable facts (and other data) from which the directions, hopes, and goals are determined. There is little room for guessing in planned change, such as, "I think . . . let's try." One kind of data gathering that was popularized at the Institute for Social Research (also at the University of Michigan, the hub of planned change and OD in the 1960s) is called survey research. (More will be said about this in the next section, "Phases of OD.") The key to planned change is *acknowledging* a problem, a growth goal, or concern, and *understanding* the need for the change.

A somewhat more sophisticated model of planned change draws upon Lewin's view of the change process (see Fig. 8-1). In this case, the four elements in the above theory have been expanded and differentiated. The identified components are those most often alluded to and followed by individuals carrying out significant planned change efforts.

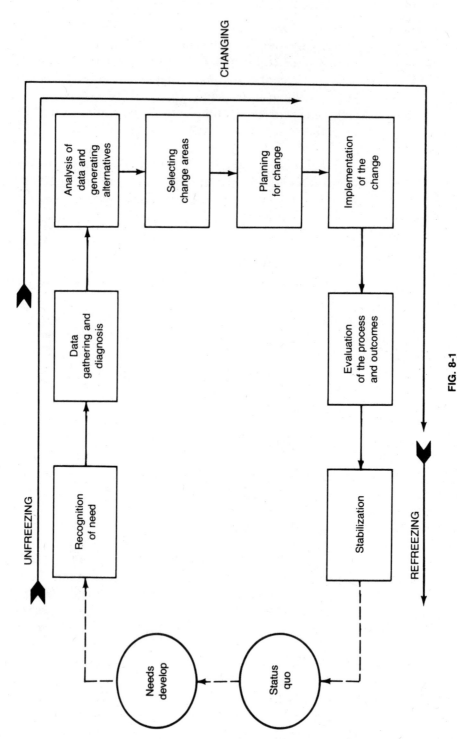

FIG. 8-1

The process of change and steps in planned change.

Principles of change

Over the past 40 years many hypotheses and generalizations about change have been offered. These are concepts or theories that when explored and implemented by those involved will facilitate constructive change. Unfortunately, it is common to operate from some principles of change that are entirely unfounded. Below are six misconceptions about change that must be dispelled before successful change can occur:

1. It is natural and inevitable for people to resist change.
2. One training workshop is likely to bring about significant organizational changes.
3. Using personal appeal increases acceptance of a change.
4. Change within a work group has little effect on other parts of the organization.
5. It is not important that organization leaders be involved with changes initiated by work groups.
6. As long as employees have satisfactorily expressed their views about an organization change, it is not always necessary to feed information back to employees.

Presented on p. 244 is a definitive list of substantiated principles of change. It goes beyond the scope of this chapter to present supporting research or other documentation for these principles. Readers desiring such input are encouraged to explore the literature for corroboration.

Resistance to change

"Resistance to change is not inevitable. People may fear it as a threat to their security and their way of doing things. On the other hand, the idea of change can also produce pleasant anticipation of new experiences and beliefs."[15] Much of change historically has been forced on systems. Under such conditions, change and changing have been met with high degrees of resistance. It is this resistance that planned change researchers and theorists began to explore in the 1950s. Under what specific conditions do people resist change? Kurt Lewin, Alvin Zander, and Dorwin Cartwright provided the most significant data in their pioneering research efforts. It is their findings that prompted many of the phases and characteristics for successful planned change activities. Their conclusions are presented on p. 245. People want to grow and want to develop (see Chapter 4). Therefore, it is imperative that change activities support the growth process. Most significantly, growing (changing) takes time. Change that does not take into consideration the element of time is likely to experience a high degree of resistance.

Timing must flow in conjunction with the natural growth process, no matter how fast or slow. In organizational settings, growth and timing relationships are compounded because of the number of animate and inanimate

CHANGE PRINCIPLES

1. **PRINCIPLE OF INTERDEPENDENCE**

   A system has many interrelated parts; a change in one part affects other parts or other systems.

2. **PRINCIPLE OF HOMEOSTASIS**

   Change upsets a system's equilibrium, so it may be resisted. Change must be reinforced or the system will revert to old patterns.

3. **PRINCIPLE OF PARTICIPATION**

   Persons affected by a change should participate in making the change.

4. **PRINCIPLE OF ACCURATE DIAGNOSING**

   An accurate diagnosis ensures a change plan aimed at the right target.

5. **PRINCIPLE OF OPPOSING FORCES**

   Change agents must know how to analyze and manage the forces operating for and against a change.

6. **PRINCIPLE OF PROPER TIMING**

   The time should be "ripe" for introducing a change.

7. **PRINCIPLE OF FLEXIBILITY**

   Change agents and change plans need built-in adaptability.

8. **PRINCIPLE OF INEVITABLE CONFLICT**

   Conflict may occur at any step in the planned change process.

9. **PRINCIPLE OF SELF-UNDERSTANDING**

   Change agents need to know themselves and use this knowledge in planning for change.

variables involved: people, departments, policies and procedures, the organization, informal groups, persons external to the system. Resistance to change is not inevitable. However, because people's support is requisite to change goals, certain activities must be avoided and others must be implemented.

Acceptance of change

Planned change founders had a commitment not to limit their efforts to "what not to do." For that reason, much work has been carried out over the last 20 years to identify those characteristics that will increase the likelihood that people will accept an organizational change. Listed on p. 245 are those conditions that, if implemented, will increase acceptance of change while actu-

RESISTANCE TO CHANGE IN ORGANIZATIONS: SOME CAUSES

1. The change is not specified through documentation.
2. The purpose for the change has not been clarified or substantiated.
3. People affected by the change have not been involved in the planning for change.
4. Personal appeal has been a primary strategy utilized to gain acceptance for a change.
5. Work group's operations and patterns have been disregarded.
6. Employees have not been kept informed about change.
7. Employees' worries and concerns about possible failure have not been explored or allayed.
8. Excessive work pressure is created during the implementation phase of the change.
9. Issues regarding job security and concomitant anxiety have not been attended to in open, real ways.

PEOPLE WILL ACCEPT AN ORGANIZATIONAL CHANGE
IF THEY ARE . . .

1. Involved in the process of change
2. Asked to contribute (knowledge, attitudes, suggestions, feelings, opinions) to the change
3. Informed of the reasons for and advantages of the change—especially as they relate to issues of uncertainty and anxiety about the change
4. Communicated with honestly in all facets of the change*
5. Given concrete and specific feedback about the change*
6. Respected for their feelings, whether supportive or opposed to the change
7. Asked and given what assistance is needed to deal with the effects of the change on the job
8. Recognized appropriately for their specific contributions to the implementation of the change

*These two requirements tend to create an atmosphere of confidence and trust in and of themselves.

ally enhancing the change. Perhaps the most fundamental of these conditions is the one that focuses on involvement. This has been the single most significant factor in assuring the acceptance and active support of an organizational change. In the last 10 years, the concept of *participative* management has been advocated and honed as the style most conducive to organizational and personal well-being. Buying into the concept of participation is necessary to such strategies as quality circles, theory Z, human resources development, team building, and organizational development. It is the investment of time and resources in learning and putting into operation participative theory and strategies that often dissuades organizations from realizing their hopes, goals, and needs. Leaders are willing to justify the expenditure of resources for quality circles or team-building programs or even organizational development; they are less comfortable, however, with verbalizing such expenditures on "participative management." This is unfortunate because nearly all of today's real innovations vis-à-vis change and organizational survival require this foundation.

The component of change that is most appropriate to this chapter is the participative process. Represented below are assumptions underlying this relationship. Before people learn *how* to be participative, they must have the opportunity to explore and come to grips with these assumptions. It is adherence to these assumptions that will distinguish obvious tokenism from programs deeply rooted in the mutual commitment to organization and people. As a reader about to embark on some organizational change, take a moment to read the assumptions and decide "where you are" on each assumption (from agree to disagree). Research supports agreeing; perhaps this is a place for you to start—for you to have opportunity to grow.

Readiness

An important variable in the acceptance of a change is that of readiness. What is currently the state of the system being considered for change? Forc-

---

CHANGE:
ASSUMPTIONS UNDERLYING THE PARTICIPATIVE PROCESS

- Persons to be affected by plans and decisions should have a part in making these plans and decisions.
- Such involvement leads to an investment of interest, time, and responsibility on the part of the participants.
- This procedure assumes the selection of realistic goals.
- It is a way of working *toward* something rather than getting away from problems.
- The brainstorming phases stimulate creativity through the nonjudgmental, free atmosphere.
- There is no preconceived way of reaching the goals.
- There is an emphasis on alternatives all the way through the process: alternative views, goals, and action plans.
- Because the work is done in group settings, there is much opportunity to build on each other's ideas and to develop collaboration.
- There is orderly movement from imagining, to goal selection, to diagnosing the forces in the field, to beginning initial action steps.

ing change will not work if cost effectiveness and improved organizational efficiency are major criteria and goals for the change. Those involved in the change must not move before people or systems involved are ready. The first step is to determine each variable's state of readiness. Assuming is no substitute for knowing: "They'll never go for it" or "That's the way it's going to be done no matter what we do" are no substitutes for quantifiable data that demonstrate: "This is where each system is." These latter data can be used as the basis to build readiness development programs—the first step.

There are five factors to assess when considering the readiness of an organization. Organizations must determine the status of each of these factors:

1. *Desire to improve.* People must want to change.
2. *Realization of need.* People must be aware of the need for change.
3. *Acceptable climate.* The organization must provide the opportunity and must continually demonstrate its willingness to support positive change.
4. *Need for feedback.* People must know that their input will be sought and utilized.
5. *Reward for improvements.* People must believe their efforts will be rewarded.

Another way to explore organizational readiness is in terms of "A Diagnostic Model for Organizational Change" developed by Steven Ruma and Kenneth Sole (see Fig. 8-2).[26] Utilizing a quadrant design, they explore readiness in terms of functionality and fixedness. Quadrant I represents those aspects or parts of the organization that are functioning at optimal levels and that are amenable to change when necessary. As circumstances arise, change is possible and can be readily implemented. Examples are a building with room for expansion or a well-trained board of directors (problem solving,

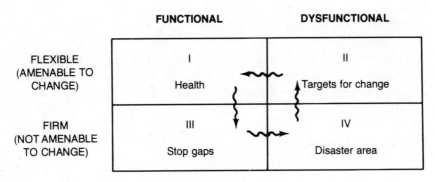

FIG. 8-2

A diagnostic model for organizational change. (Reproduced by special permission from Ruma, S.J.: Social change—ideas and applications: A diagnostic model for organizational change, NTL Institute **4**(4):16, 1974.)

group membership) that is willing to examine its own processes. Quadrant II represents the area most likely for the implementation of planned change. These aspects of the organization are dysfunctional (they are not working well), but they are open to change. Common aspects include organizational norms for reward and punishment, modes of communication, and job functions and responsibilities. Quadrant III usually consists of temporary means of dealing with problems; they may be effective in the short run but will not be so in the long run. An overdependence on this stopgap strategy will be just as dangerous to the organization as relying on a temporary solution for dealing with one specific incidence. Examples of quadrant III variables include "acting directors," temporary buildings, or technology that is narrow in its application. Quadrant IV is, as Ruma describes, the area of "organizational disaster." It comprises those aspects of the system that at present are neither effective nor amenable to change. They must be acknowledged, but their existence must not be overrated. The best ways to work in these areas are to institute activities that limit the spread of negative effects and avoid the wastage of valuable resources and energy on them.

In using this model, step 1 is quadrant I. Identifying the healthy aspects of the organization tends to provoke minimal anxiety; it points out what is being done well to use as a general ideal for further action, and it allows working comfort with the quadrant concept. It also reinforces the continued utilization of time, energy, and support of these aspects. Step 2 is the listing and prioritizing, according to "readiness to be changed," of factors relevant to quadrant II. Note that prioritizing is based on readiness and not "need to change" in terms of time, costs, or energy. Organizations that decide to work on factors based on need to change criteria irrespective of readiness may become frustrated and disappointed. This activity clearly helps identify the source of these feelings. Goals for change should be matched with both *affective* and *energy* readiness. Items in quadrants III and IV are listed, but not focused on. It helps organization members to be aware of these factors vis-à-vis their dysfunctionality.

A primary reason for determining readiness is to provide interventions that will minimize resistance as well as the likelihood of failure. Preparing organizational elements for success will create a firm base of support and stability crucial during periods of change. The following elements are considered primary:

- Management systems
- Technical support
- Administrative systems
- Quality systems
- Training and development systems
- Feedback and recognition systems
- Bargaining units (formal or informal)

The most commonly utilized method of determining readiness is through asking questions in somewhat structured ways such as questionnaires, meetings, interviews, and informal observations. More will be said about these methods in a later section under the topic "Organizational Clarification— Where Are We?" Suffice it to say here that at this stage of change, determining readiness and knowing where and how to start are most important. A false step can reverse or undermine the much-needed change activity. Other dimensions to assess for readiness may include the following:

- Policies
- Organization commitment
- Training and development
- Employee work cycle
- Performance
- Data management

Again, for an organization to initiate change, it must be ready. Another method of determining readiness is to assume readiness upon completion of the following three activities in the order presented:

1. Analysis of current and future human resource requirements
2. Development of an internal support system that provides sound performance management programs
3. Development of a highly functional internal communications system that relies on both systemwide and one-to-one communications, whether written or verbal.

The change agent and ethics

One of the most meaningful contributions made by planned change theorists and practitioners has to do with the ethics of change. Although a later section of this chapter fully expands on the change agent concept—role, skills, knowledge base, and functions—the concept of ethics is discussed here in light of the change agent's expertise. In the 1950s and 1960s the excellent research and theory building that occurred regarding change brought to the surface an assumption or concern that virtually any change might be implemented utilizing the principles and findings described in this chapter. It placed a massive burden on the parents of planned change. What was acceptable change? Who had the right to determine the change? It was their commitment to ethical resolution of these questions that led them to concentrate on the issue and its ramifications for agents of change.

Planned change and organizational development efforts require expertise in the process of change. In the 1960s that requirement was translated into a person—a change agent—who had change agentry skills and knowledge. One of their earliest and most profound questions was: "What change do we implement?" After years of work, change agents unequivocally state that for change to be truly effective (i.e., long lasting, productive, enhancing), it must "fit the system" in which it is to occur. It must be congruent with the system's values, goals, climate, activities, and people. Changes instigated that do not take organizational fit into consideration will result in loss—of people, of time, of dollars, of prestige, of clients. It is for this reason that so many of the efforts toward reducing nurse turnover have failed miserably to date; the change strategy has not fit the goals, climate, values, and people of the facility. It is "someone else's solution" and it *cannot* be imposed and cannot work in another system. The implications for change agents are clear: it is not their job to come into an organization and institute change *they think is best*. Rather, their job is (1) to facilitate the organization identifying change areas for itself and (2) to help organization members understand the principles and processes of change so *they* can apply them to the organization. It also becomes the change agent's task to educate members vis-à-vis requisite skills for bringing about and managing change efforts. These types of change agent activities are more time consuming but more contributory to actual resolution of organizational concerns; they also allow the organization to retain the expertise for future endeavors.

The first ethical dilemma was "solved" with the recognition that people to be affected by the change had to determine the directions for and goals of the change. The second ethical dilemma faced by change agents has to do with "Who should carry out the change?" This concern on the surface tends to be less an issue for the organization than for the change agent. That is because change agents have learned that for successful change to occur, the people affected by the change must be involved in the implementation phases of the change. The change agent might implement organization-determined changes and then leave. These changes, however, will not stay in place in the long run. It is therefore imperative that change agents agree to facilitate those change efforts that include those persons whose activities will be altered by the change. To do otherwise would be pretentious and ineffective. To do otherwise would not in the long run benefit the organization. In fact, it often is harmful to the system.

A third ethical dilemma faced by change agents has to do with confidentiality. Change—no matter how large or small—has a great impact on people. It touches their values, their hopes, their strengths and limitations, their attitudes, and their own sense of worth. Given this response in people, combined with the highly developed interpersonal skills, the true concern, and the nonjudgmental perspective of the change agent, people tend to deal with their reactions. They tend to do this by sharing and talking with the change agent. As a result the change agent is privy to massive amounts of information. It is this opportunity to share and the process of sharing that are most effective in organizational members' acceptance of change. The data gleaned from these interactions are far less important than the interaction itself. Therefore, it is not worth jeopardizing trust and an effective, giving relationship for the sake of telling others what someone said or feels. To a lesser extent, the same kind of "telling" by a change agent of his or her observations with those not involved in the activities being commented on is easily as harmful. For both the person(s) and the organization, confidentiality is imperative. It is, however, not an easy matter for the change agent. This person must process and keep a great deal of information, of emotion, of responsibility. It is for this reason that collegiality and networking have been so important to the profession; the change agent needs someone to share with who understands, who is safe, and who can help explore the data for the purpose of helping people. More is said about this in the section, "The People in OD." It is enough to say that confidentiality is difficult but that a professional change agent is one who is committed to it and who develops mechanisms for self to assure it.

It is this history of ethical dilemma combined with day-to-day experiences that drive home the importance of being ethical. It is being ethical that has prompted *the confrontation of ethical concerns to become a normative process* for agents of change. One of their first and primary considerations has to do with ethics: for themselves, their relationships, and client systems and their subparts. Few other professions have focused on ethics more intently in their daily activity and service than change agents. There is an ethical component in every change. Change agents legitimize the exploration and implications of ethics as part of their contribution to organization enhancement. It is perhaps in putting into operation "dealing with ethics in all phases of change" that early planned change experts made their greatest inroads. Change agents now have the tools and theoretical support to proceed ethically *and* productively with organizational change.

PHASES OF OD

Although much new knowledge resulted from the work of planned change researchers and practitioners, there was no "whole" from which to operate—no thread that tied all of these findings together. Pseudo-change experts began utilizing the stages of planned change in consulting or managerial applications without using its soul—that is, the depth of knowledge regarding change discussed in the first section, "The Process of Change." Both of these factors led to the initiation of a new body of knowledge, of educational strategy called organizational development (OD).*

What is OD?

Perhaps the best way to conceptualize OD is to offer a variety of definitions.

*Note: organizational development, *not* organization development. The latter refers to skills and activities that focus on organization improvement, usually irrespective of human resource development or involvement; it tends to focus on the major functional areas of systems (e.g., finance, accounting, administration, marketing) and their responsibilities and interrelationships.

Michael McGill. Organizational Development is a conscious, planned process of developing an organization's capabilities so that it can attain and sustain an optimum level of performance as measured by efficiency, effectiveness, and health. Operationally, OD is a normative process of addressing the questions: "Where are we?" "Where do we want to be?" "How do we get from where we are to where we want to be?" This process is undertaken by members of the organization using a variety of techniques, often in collaboration with a behavioral science consultant.[18]

Delbert Fisher. Organizational Development stresses the involvement of staff members in improving organizational effectiveness. It is an evolving collection of philosophies, concepts, and techniques aimed at improving an organization's performance. It is an intervention that involves members of the organization in identifying their own creative resources, diagnosing problems, developing alternative solutions, and providing a mechanism for continual self-renewal.[8]

Warren Bennis. Organizational Development is an educational strategy employing the widest possible means of experience-based behavior in order to achieve more and better organizational choices in a highly turbulent world.[4]

James Gibson et al. Organizational Development is a planned process of reeducation and training designed to facilitate organizational adaptation to changing environmental demands.[9]

Michael Beer. Organizational Development is a broad framework for understanding a variety of organizational problems and a variety of approaches and methods for organizational improvement. It has a unique tendency to emphasize a collaborative process of diagnosis and change and to search for innovative structures and processes for dealing with traditional organizational problems.[2]

Warner Burke. Organizational Development is a planned sustained effort to change an organization's culture (e.g., behavioral norms: organization purpose, policies, values; channels of communication; centers and modes of influence; and climate).[6]

Warner Burke. Organizational Development is a process for developing an organization climate based on social science principles for diagnosing and coping with inadequacies in interpersonal, group, and intergroup behavior in the organization's culture (normative system, structure, work flow patterns). The process leads to behavior changes in formal decision making, communication, planning, problem solving, and the exercise of authority and responsibility. O.D. focuses also on improving and reinforcing existing strengths of the organization.[7]

Although implied, the one major element that must be a part of any definition of OD is its commitment to identifying processes, activities, methodologies, and constructs that are organization specific. Organizational development is well suited to meeting the challenges of the contemporary work world (e.g., productivity, employee commitment, and organizational adaptation). It is, however, the "fit" of the processes to each separate organization that separates OD from other improvement strategies. It is committed to congruence in all facets of its definition and action.

Organizational development is a process that is appropriate to any organization no matter what its state. In their classic article, "Crises in a Developing Organization," Lippitt and Schmidt[16] recognized three major developmental stages of organizations: birth, youth, and maturity. They then identified critical concerns, key issues, and consequences of not meeting the concerns relevant to each stage (see Table 8-2). Given this perspective, organizations are constantly facing new demands: growth begets growth. The implications are clear: with each stage of OD a separate knowledge base and set of executive-managerial skills and attitudes are required (see Table 8-3). It is this natural progression of the organization and its management leadership that OD efforts facilitate and that OD *naturally* addresses.

Organizational development is especially applicable to service organizations that are people intensive such as hospitals—that is, that rely heavily on their employees for continued effectiveness. Because OD improves organization effectiveness, it is an ideal strategy for today's hospitals. These hospitals are faced with budget restrictions, personnel cutbacks, technological advances, and public demand for quality. In terms of this book, the OD intervention is most relevant to retaining staff nurses, the primary service givers in

TABLE 8-2
Stages of organizational development

Developmental stage	Critical concern	Key issues	Consequences if concern is not met
Birth	1. To create a new organization	What to risk	Frustration and inaction
	2. To survive as a viable system	What to sacrifice	Death of organization; further subsidy by "faith" capital
Youth	3. To gain stability	How to organize	Reactive, crisis-dominated organization; opportunistic rather than self-directing attitudes and policies
	4. To gain reputation and develop pride	How to review and evaluate	Difficulty in attracting good personnel and clients; inappropriate, overly aggressive, and distorted image building
Maturity	5. To achieve uniqueness and adaptability	Whether and how to change	Unnecessarily defensive or competitive attitudes; diffusion of energy; loss of most creative personnel
	6. To contribute to society	Whether and how to share	Possible lack of public respect and appreciation; bankruptcy or profit loss

Reprinted by permission from Lippitt, G., and Schmidt, W.H.: Crisis in a developing organization, Harvard Bus. Rev. 45(6):102-112, Nov.-Dec. 1967. Copyright © 1967 by the President and Fellows of Harvard College. All rights reserved.

the hospital. The reason OD is most appropriate for improving retention is that its underlying behavioral assumptions are congruent with the prerequisites for nurse retention. These include the following:

1. Attitudes most employees have toward work and their work habits are usually more reactions to the work environment and how they are treated, than they are intrinsic personality characteristics of the individual. Efforts to change attitudes should be directed toward changing how the person is treated rather than trying to change the person.

TABLE 8-3
Requirements to meet the need for organizational change at various levels of organizational maturity

Critical concern	Knowledge	Skills	Attitude
To create a system	Clearly perceived short-range objective in mind of top manager	Ability to transmit knowledge into action by self and into orders to others	Belief in own ability, product, market
To survive	The short-range objectives that need to be communicated	Communications know-how; ability to adjust to changing conditions	Faith in future
To stabilize	How top manager can predict relevant factors and make long-range plans	Ability to transmit planning knowledge into communicable objectives	Trust in other members of organization
To earn a good reputation	Planning know-how and understanding of goals on part of whole executive team	Facility of allowing others a voice in decision making, involving others in decision making and obtaining commitments from them, and communicating objectives to customers	Interest in customers/clients
To achieve uniqueness	Understanding on part of policy team of how others should set own objectives, and of how to manage subunits of the organization	Ability to teach others to plan, proficiency in integrating plans of subunits into objectives and resources of organization	Self-confidence
To earn respect and appreciation	General management understanding of the larger objectives of organization and of society	Ability to apply own organization and resources to the problems of the larger community	Sense of responsibility to society and mankind

2. Work organized to meet the employee's needs as well as to achieve organizational goals leads to greater productivity and high quality.
3. Most individuals seek challenging work and desire responsibility for accomplishing goals to which they are committed.
4. The group not the individual is the basic unit of change.
5. Expressing feelings is an important part of becoming committed to decision or task. The climate in most organizations tends to suppress feelings and thus reduce commitment to task.
6. Relationships that are open, supportive, and trusting facilitate individual growth in a group.
7. Commitment to change is more effectively obtained when everyone involved participates actively in planning and implementing the change.[28]

Organizational development is a strategy most often utilized because it confronts the particular issues of contemporary organization life. Although we are focusing here on only one of these issues for hospital organizations, the retention of staff nurses, the application of OD is a total organization methodology and is most often implemented as such. Though it can be applied narrowly (e.g., to nurse retention), it will have organizational impact far beyond that concern. The reason for OD's broadly based applicability is evident in the goals of OD (see list below). No other statement or process more effectively ties together organizational and human enhancement.

GOALS OF ORGANIZATIONAL DEVELOPMENT*

1. To create an open, problem-solving climate.
2. To supplement the authority associated with role or status with the authority of knowledge and competence.
3. To locate decision-making and problem-solving responsibilities as close to the information source as possible.
4. To build trust among persons and groups throughout an organization.
5. To make competition more relevant to work goals and to maximize collaborative efforts.
6. To develop a reward system which recognizes both the achievement of the organization's goals (profits or service) and development of people.
7. To increase the sense of "ownership" of organization objectives throughout the work force.
8. To help managers to manage according to relevant objectives rather than according to "past practices" or according to objectives which do not make sense for one's areas of responsibilities.
9. To increase self-direction for people within the organization.

---

*Hampton, David R., and Hardison, Nancy M.: *Contemporary management (instructor's manual)*, New York, 1981, McGraw-Hill Book Co.

Applied OD is the cyclical implementation of seven phases. The remainder of this section is devoted to the identification, description, and activities of each of these phases.*

A flowchart representing the cyclical process of OD as defined here is presented in Fig. 8-3. It begins, ends, continues with organizational clarification. The time line of the OD process is not predetermined—it is ongoing.

Phase I, Part A: Organizational clarification—Who are we?

The primary purpose of this phase is to verbalize the organization's missions, goals, membership, and history. The attempt is made to pull together the myriad of perspectives and forces contributing to the definition of "who we are." This phase usually occurs in a retreat setting often lasting for as long as a week. Participants include the OD consultant(s) who has been chosen to facilitate the process, executive leadership of the organization, and significant other representatives (hereafter referred to as the task force). The group size should not be unwieldy but should not omit anyone key to organizational growth. While organization members focus on the sharing and clarification of perceptions and data, the OD consultant(s) designs and facilitates the process in such a way as to increase the comfortable transition to the next phase and to returning to back-home tasks.† Although a retreat may suffice, the exact length of phase IA is determined by the current state of the organization, the breadth and depth of its intentions, and its progress during the off-site portion. A work-place follow-up session(s) is crucial before moving to phase IB. The consultant's responsibility, further, is to help the group translate its recognition of "who we are" to consensus. Finally, during this phase the OD consultant's job is to help the group identify the criteria for defining productivity vis-à-vis OD; the participants are encouraged to utilize those criteria that are appropriate to their organization.‡ "Who are we?" The organization, the members of that organization, the retreat participants as persons and as role representatives, and the OD consultant.

---

*Caution: A complete discussion regarding OD is impossible within the confines and purpose of this chapter and book. The intent in presenting the phases, concepts, and methodologies is to supplement or pave the way for a meaningful OD effort. It is meant to familiarize hospital leadership with a most appropriate intervention for its development. The bibliography at the end of this chapter provides many sound resources for expanding the reader's knowledge of and confidence in organizational development.

†The consultant builds into the design or has readily available a variety of tools, theories, concepts, and activities that broaden the scope of the defining "Who are we." Simplistic characterizations and sharing are usually not appropriate to this phase. Clarification of the necessity and elements of hard work related to OD is carefully examined.

‡A further task of the consultant is to define terms and activities common to OD. It is this person's responsibility to educate. This is usually done in conjunction with the activities undertaken during Phase IA and IB (and throughout for that matter) by labeling and examining the activities being experienced.

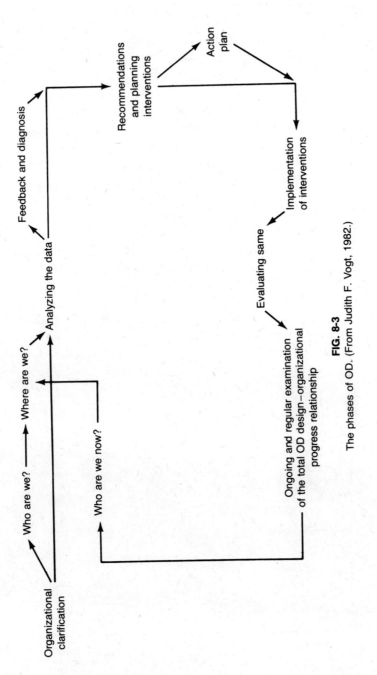

FIG. 8-3

The phases of OD. (From Judith F. Vogt, 1982.)

Phase I, Part B: Organizational clarification—Where are we?

Once a group has determined and clarified for itself who it is, the next developmental step is to determine "Where it is." The persons who participated in Phase I have by now become a separate entity. They are, however, to be conceived of, for themselves and for the organization and its membership, as a representative mirror of the organization—as the OD task force. During the initial part of Phase IA, this group begins to define its purpose, its loyalties, its potential, and criteria for success and failure. This step is important because its focus is now the organization; before this the individual members probably had a more limited focus. Time must be allowed and activities must be implemented that assure this transition; new norms and definitions and methods of accomplishment must be identified. Just as this group is determining "Where are we?", it must also learn "where the organization is." (In OD there tends to be a direct relationship between the development of the organization and the development of the OD task force.) To do this it gathers data.

Data gathering is the crux of OD. Before expanding on this process, a note of caution is in order. Organizations must not gather or seek out any data on which they do not intend to take action. Figure 8-4 graphically explores the long-range consequences on productivity of collecting and ignoring the information. Succinctly, organizational productivity will fall below its original level if action is not forthcoming. Data gathering brings discontent to the surface so it can be confronted and eliminated. If it is not acted on in this man-

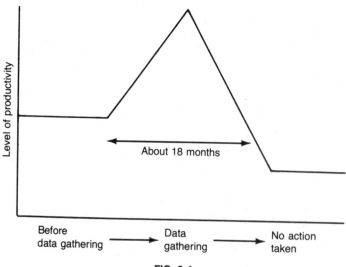

FIG. 8-4
Impact on productivity of not taking action on data collected during Phase II.

ner, it will erupt and cause intense stress on the organization, resulting in inefficiency and lowered productivity.

The first step in this data-gathering process is to generate the overall design. Included in this design are the following elements:

1. The groups and content on which to gather assessment data are determined (e.g., "What are the significant variables at which we need to look?"). Robert Johnston[13] has identified internal and external subsystem variables that may potentially be examined; these are presented in chart form in Table 8-4. Collecting data on each of these areas can be a massive project requiring up to a year to accomplish. Usually, organizations choose "starting places" based on existing qualitative data. Still, Johnston's framework is an invaluable resource to organizations who are involved in OD.

An uncomplicated but highly effective model for gathering information is presented on p. 261. In this model, six functional areas are perceived as basic to answering the question, "Where are we?": soundness of human relations, soundness of organization structure, management effectiveness, efficient work methods, quality of personnel practices, and soundness of union-management (or employee-management) relations. Some typical questions for exploring each area are presented in the list on p. 261, on which the organization is encouraged to expand.

One possible tool for gathering data about one specific group, management, is presented on pp. 262-264. This particular instrument is especially meaningful if respondents are encouraged to participate in dialogue about their reactions, comments, and views regarding each area. One area often overlooked in the data-gathering phase is physical setting. Fritz Steele,[29] in his book, *Physical Settings and Organizational Development*, clearly portrays the effect that physical surroundings have on performance, attitudes toward job, and organization. Employee attitudes and effectiveness can be altered and improved through the careful design of their physical settings. Seeking input on positive sources of satisfaction is more important than what to eliminate. Organizations are encouraged to consider this variable when determining what information is to be gathered.

2. Clarification of the types of survey research methodologies to be utilized ("How do we gather the data?")—for example, climate survey, attitudinal survey, individual and group interviews, hard data search, paper-and-pencil questionnaires, open-ended or closed instrumentation—is necessary. One of the most authoritative resources for this phase is David Nadler's book, *Feedback and Organizational Development: Using Data-Based Methods*.[22] Many OD consultants have the book as required reading before implementing Phase II. The data-gathering methods chosen must fit the persons or areas about which information is sought.

3. Who will gather what data and how will it be disseminated throughout

Text continued on p. 264.

TABLE 8-4
Subsystems that influence organization system outputs*

Internal subsystems								External subsystems		Whole organization subsystem
Individual subsystem	+	Social subsystem	+	Operation subsystem	+	Administration subsystem	+	Client or demand subsystem	=	
Attitudes		Climate		Work flow		Policy		Customer satisfaction		(Output variables)
Self-image		Status role		Equipment		Wage-Salary		Service to and reactions to users		Profit/loss service
Skills: social technical		Decision-making management style		Location: physical environment		Promotions, fringe benefits		Constraints-Taxes		Costs, attendance
Life values		Values		Material		Hiring and firing		Laws and regulations		Turnover
Behavior		Communication		Work arrangements		Raises		Competition		Commitment
Goals: job, career		Work team goals		Schedules		Budgets Reporting		Mass media and publics Labor		Involvement
Self-appraisal		Progress review				Auditing		Government (state, local, federal), international factors		Motivation Quality

*A revision and expansion of Dyer's model (1976), by Robert W. Johnston.[13]

TYPICAL QUESTIONS IN THE SIX FUNCTIONAL AREAS

HOW SOUND ARE THE HUMAN RELATIONS?

What are people doing to each other?
What are the people doing for each other?
Do members of the group believe in the purpose of the organization?
Do they believe in the leadership?
Do they communicate and participate effectively?
Do they believe in the company?

HOW SOUND IS THE ORGANIZATION STRUCTURE?

Does it work effectively?
How does the informal organization (the informal personal relationships and their use as the means for the functioning of the department) conform to the formal organization?
What kinds of informal subgroups or cliques have been formed?
What marked splits are there between various levels of management or between management and employees?
What is the social hierarchy and what are the status symbols?
Do people understand and accept the organization structure, lines of command, and delegation of authority and responsibility?
Do individuals have an opportunity to use their initiative to demonstrate their ability and to grow?

HOW EFFECTIVE IS THE MANAGEMENT?

Is there any evidence of planning?
How effectively do the executives direct, delegate, and coordinate?
Do they initiate effective action and work with others on a basis of mutuality?
Are they concerned about developing people?
Do people know where they stand as far as their superiors are concerned?

HOW EFFICIENT ARE THE WORK METHODS?

Are the executives' methods conscious and economy minded?
Are the procedures organized or disorganized?
Are there any written instructions?

WHAT IS THE QUALITY OF PERSONNEL PRACTICES?

How are individuals selected and promoted?
How are they evaluated and trained?
Do their pay rates correspond to the levels of work?
Are they kept informed about company matters?

ARE THE UNION-MANAGEMENT RELATIONS SOUND?

What is the attitude toward the contract?
What are the attitudes toward the union representatives?
Are the union rules being followed in spirit as well as in word?
Are the rules understood?

AN ASSESSMENT TOOL FOR MANAGEMENT

INSTRUCTIONS

On the following pages will be listed several characteristics or qualities connected with your management position. For each such characteristic, you will be asked to give three ratings:

 a. *How much* of the characteristic is there *now* connected with your management position?

 b. *How much* of the characteristic do you think *should be* connected with your management position?

 c. *How important* is this position characteristic *to you?*

For each of the *13* items, answer *all 3* questions by circling the number on the rating scale.

        (minimum)   1   2   3   4   5   6   7   (maximum)

On the scale, low numbers represent low or minimum amounts, and high numbers represent high or maximum amounts.

Date _____

1. The *prestige* of my management position *outside* the company (that is, the regard received from others *not* in the company):
    a. How much is there now?
       (minimum)   1   2   3   4   5   6   7   (maximum)
    b. How much should there be?
       (minimum)   1   2   3   4   5   6   7   (maximum)
    c. How important is this to me?
       (minimum)   1   2   3   4   5   6   7   (maximum)

2. The *opportunity*, in my management position, for *participation in the determination of methods and procedures:*
    a. How much is there now?
       (minimum)   1   2   3   4   5   6   7   (maximum)
    b. How much should there be?
       (minimum)   1   2   3   4   5   6   7   (maximum)
    c. How important is this to me?
       (minimum)   1   2   3   4   5   6   7   (maximum)

3. The *feeling of security* in my management position:
    a. How much is there now?
       (minimum)   1   2   3   4   5   6   7   (maximum)
    b. How much should there be?
       (minimum)   1   2   3   4   5   6   7   (maximum)
    c. How important is this to me?
       (minimum)   1   2   3   4   5   6   7   (maximum)

4. The *feeling of worthwhile accomplishment* in my management position:
    a. How much is there now?
       (minimum)   1   2   3   4   5   6   7   (maximum)

  b. How much should there be?
    (minimum)   1   2   3   4   5   6   7   (maximum)
  c. How important is this to me?
    (minimum)   1   2   3   4   5   6   7   (maximum)
5. The *opportunity for independent thought and action* in my management position:
  a. How much is there now?
    (minimum)   1   2   3   4   5   6   7   (maximum)
  b. How much should there be?
    (minimum)   1   2   3   4   5   6   7   (maximum)
  c. How important is this to me?
    (minimum)   1   2   3   4   5   6   7   (maximum)
6. The *feeling of self-esteem* a person gets from being in my management position:
  a. How much is there now?
    (minimum)   1   2   3   4   5   6   7   (maximum)
  b. How much should there be?
    (minimum)   1   2   3   4   5   6   7   (maximum)
  c. How important is this to me?
    (minimum)   1   2   3   4   5   6   7   (maximum)
7. The *opportunity to develop close friendships* in my management position:
  a. How much is there now?
    (minimum)   1   2   3   4   5   6   7   (maximum)
  b. How much should there be?
    (minimum)   1   2   3   4   5   6   7   (maximum)
  c. How important is this to me?
    (minimum)   1   2   3   4   5   6   7   (maximum)
8. The *opportunity for personal growth and development* in my management position:
  a. How much is there now?
    (minimum)   1   2   3   4   5   6   7   (maximum)
  b. How much should there be?
    (minimum)   1   2   3   4   5   6   7   (maximum)
  c. How important is this to me?
    (minimum)   1   2   3   4   5   6   7   (maximum)
9. The opportunity, in my management position, for *participation in the setting of goals:*
  a. How much is there now?
    (minimum)   1   2   3   4   5   6   7   (maximum)
  b. How much should there be?
    (minimum)   1   2   3   4   5   6   7   (maximum)
  c. How important is this to me?
    (minimum)   1   2   3   4   5   6   7   (maximum)

Continued.

AN ASSESSMENT TOOL FOR MANAGEMENT—cont'd

10. The *prestige* of my management position *inside* the company (that is, the regard received from others *in* the company):
    a. How much is there now?
    (minimum)   1   2   3   4   5   6   7   (maximum)
    b. How much should there be?
    (minimum)   1   2   3   4   5   6   7   (maximum)
    c. How important is this to me?
    (minimum)   1   2   3   4   5   6   7   (maximum)

11. The opportunity, in my management position, *to give help to other people:*
    a. How much is there now?
    (minimum)   1   2   3   4   5   6   7   (maximum)
    b. How much should there be?
    (minimum)   1   2   3   4   5   6   7   (maximum)
    c. How important is this to me?
    (minimum)   1   2   3   4   5   6   7   (maximum)

12. The *authority* connected with my management position:
    a. How much is there now?
    (minimum)   1   2   3   4   5   6   7   (maximum)
    b. How much should there be?
    (minimum)   1   2   3   4   5   6   7   (maximum)
    c. How important is this to me?
    (minimum)   1   2   3   4   5   6   7   (maximum)

13. The *feeling of self-fulfillment* a person gets from being in my management position (that is, the feeling of being able to use one's own unique capabilities, realizing one's potentialities):
    a. How much is there now?
    (minimum)   1   2   3   4   5   6   7   (maximum)
    b. How much should there be?
    (minimum)   1   2   3   4   5   6   7   (maximum)
    c. How important is this to me?
    (minimum)   1   2   3   4   5   6   7   (maximum)

the organization? This portion of the overall design concerns managing the OD effort. At this point, task groups and time lines are usually determined. One of the primary requirements of survey feedback methodology, which serves as the basis for OD efforts, is that the information gleaned is fed back in some useful and meaningful manner to those who provided the data. Figure 8-4 has portrayed what will happen if such a step is not undertaken. It is also to be encouraged that all respondents have the opportunity to share their reactions and insights (more is said about how this may occur in Phase II). At this point, the OD effort is transferred completely to the organization. The OD consultant now becomes truly a consultant; the organization is responsible for its direction and future. The key concept the OD expert reinforces is that *forward movement* must continue; no movement is unacceptable.

The second step in the "Where are we?" phase is materials design—that is, instrumentation. Questions such as what do we want to know, how will we use it, who will be responding, how much time do we have, and what other information will be requested from the respondents are important considerations in designing the specific tools and activities. The third and final step in Phase I is actually gathering the data—that is, implementing the overall design. All of the parameters and considerations identified during steps 1 and 2 should be carefully attended to.

Phase II: Analyzing the data—feedback and diagnosis

This phase is composed of two parts: (1) Examining the data and drawing conclusions from it; and (2) generating implications from the data and determining goals. It is during this phase that as many of the organization's human resources as are relevant to the OD goals should be involved—in seeing and analyzing the data as well as defining implications and specific goals. Again the planning and coordinating of this phase are the primary responsibilities of the OD task force formed during Phase I. The primary role of the OD consultant during this time is to help task force members determine how to present the data most effectively so that it is useful information rather than "just words" or "just numbers." One of the most effective methods for presenting data is called the force-field analysis. Discussed in depth in Chapter 4, this method helps determine the forces that support goal achievement and those that impede such achievement. Another method is to determine what data are cognitive and what data are emotional in impact (see Fig. 6-5). Analysis of this sort will help determine where and how to start toward growth (and change). Another major responsibility of the consultant is to assure that adequate time is taken on the analysis. The accuracy, thoroughness, and organization of the analysis serve as the basis for goal setting and planning. Organizational development consultants often call this phase "massaging the data"; it is an appropriate analogy, and care must be taken to allow structured as well as free-flowing diagnostic sessions.

Goal setting is the next step in Phase II. Careful attention must be paid to saying: "What do we want to accomplish now that we know who we are and where we are as an organization?" Goals based on observable data are imperative. The organization must intervene where needs exist and where the data indicate; large, unfounded jumps or gaps in feedback to goal setting can undermine the work accomplished to date. Organizational development is a step-by-step process. It respects and values this progression. This feedback-to-goal movement is an example of this characteristic.

Phase III: Recommendations and planning interventions (action plan)

This phase consists of putting into operation the goals formed in Phase II. In designing the action plan for an organization, there are really two steps. First, as many recommendations as are appropriate to the organizational circumstances–goals relationship should be identified. Second, these must be put into some justifiable whole based on certain criteria. It is at this second step that modifications of the recommendations are made to accommodate the plan and a variety of conditions. Some of the guiding considerations in designing the action plan are as follows:

1. Where and how to begin (what group, what interventions)
2. Timing and sequencing (e.g., building on skills or previous interventions)
3. Variety and types of interventions (typical interventions include organizational design changes, intergroup meetings, team building, skill-building programs—usually in communications, management development)
4. Financial latitude or limits (overall, annual considerations; return on investment potentiality; "good buy" decisions)
5. Utilization of experts
6. Innovativeness (deliberate, novel, specific change that makes goal achievement easier)
7. Degree of commitment (Who is committed and who do we want committed?)
8. Contingency plans (What do we do when we need to react—for example, in the case of resistance or when the plan is no longer appropriate?)
9. Stabilizing the system (ensuring adaptability to the system and ongoing functionality of the system as well as knowing when to rest or cease)

Literally thousands of combinations are possible in the development of the action plan. The above criteria can be utilized to increase the likelihood that the overall plan and its component parts are best for the organization. In Chapter 5, in the section on program design, additional criteria are offered for determining the makeup of the action plan. Clearly stated and agreed-on justifications should be made for both the overall plan and its parts, and these justifications should be based on task and maintenance considerations, some of which are listed below:

- Boundary maintenance and operations
- Size and territoriality

- Physical facilities
- Time use
- Goals
- Procedures
- Role definitions
- Normative beliefs and sentiments
- Structure (relationship among parts)
- Socialization methods
- Linkage with other systems

The task of the consultant is fivefold during Phase III. First, he or she asks questions that encourage further thought on both the activities and the overall plan. Second, the consultant educates the client regarding the various design considerations and elements involved in determining the psychological fit of the action plan. Third, the consultant suggests the need for utilizing expert help, possibly recommending appropriate experts as well. Fourth, the consultant encourages ongoing communications aimed at keeping the organization aware of all activities being performed vis-à-vis the assessment and data base. Whom to inform, what to inform about, how to inform, and who informs are the points in focus. This function should be incorporated into the remainder of the OD effort by a representative person or subgroup of the task force. Finally, the consultant helps the task force assess itself: its process, its progress, its strengths, its limitations. How has the task force fared in developing plans and strategies for getting work done and for effectively accomplishing objectives? How has it done to date in maintaining the organizational growth and development? This is usually carried out utilizing structured and unstructured activities. It often takes place in the original retreat setting over a 2-day period. Ample time for exploring personal and group development is imperative. The facilitator's task is to assure that broadly based analyses occur; expressions of conflict and issues of power, style, and competition/collaboration usually take precedence. Confronting rather than smoothing over is a primary consultant task. It is this activity that often prepares task force members for dealing with the reactions and consequences of Phase IV.

Phase IV: Implementation of interventions and evaluation of same

Although significant interventions into the system have already been made (e.g., task force development, data gathering and feedback, communications, asking and planning), the planned thrust is initiated during Phase IV. Common interventions include (a) management development, (b) skill training, (c) team building, (d) intergroup meetings, (e) survey feedback, (f) managing conflict, and (g) technostructural changes. Again, it is beyond the scope of this book and chapter to present the theory and to outline the component parts relevant to each of these possible focuses. A reiteration of a point made

TABLE 8-5

Organizational development matrix*

Focus	Internal subsystems			External subsystems
	Social subsystem	Technical-operation subsystem	Administration subsystem	Client or demand subsystem
Individual	Counseling Coaching Management training Testing Individual feedback Intrapersonal awareness Personal development program Management profiling Intuition development Life/career planning Management inventory	Job rotation Technical training Performance review Job enrichment Sales training	Policy-procedure analysis and change • Incentive • Hours • Promotions	Role requirements and relation- ships Distributor training Dealer training

INTEGRATED MANAGEMENT PROCESS TRAINING

Interpersonal and team	Team building, MBO Team training Team problem solving RAT (role analysis technique) Data-feedback Group diagnosis instruments Meeting engineering Process consultation T-Group	Work-flow analysis Work redesign Job enrichment Work team formation Job planning Pride of craftsman- ship project Socio-technical training VEM (viewpoint exchange meeting)	Goal setting Policy reexam- ination Motivations and control system analysis Scheduling	Open system planning Open system mapping
Intergroup and total organization	Sensing meetings Mirroring Intergroup building Confrontation conference Survey-feedback	Work systems analysis System redesign Capital equipment Improvement or development	Long-range planning Strategic planning Forecasting Budget review	Data gathering from demand systems Interface meetings with demand systems

*A revision and expansion of Dyer's model (1976), by Robert W. Johnston.[13]

TABLE 8-5—cont'd
Organizational development matrix

| Focus | Internal subsystems | | | External subsystems |
	Social subsystem	Technical-operation subsystem	Administration subsystem	Client or demand subsystem
Intergroup and total organiza- tion—cont'd	Organization diagnosis instruments Open system planning Third-party peacemaking		Analysis of information systems	Open system planning Open system mapping

earlier, however, is in order. Whatever interventions are made must be congruent with the organization's goals and stages of development. Further, it is accurate to say that most Phase IVs begin with educational programs that serve to convert potential resistance into support for the OD effort by:

1. Developing a more conducive attitude, knowledge, or skill base among organization members
2. Legitimizing time and effort spent on considering organizational issues
3. Bringing relevant organization members together to define the critical areas and issues requiring collaboration[24]

Often this takes place in some sort of interpersonnel communications skill building/OD theory base sequence. In the health care setting the second part of the sequence might include the following topics:

- Health care (organizations as open systems)
- Planning and goal setting
- Organizational design and work allocation
- Personal and managerial styles
- Roles and role clarification
- Conflict resolution: negotiation and third-party consultation
- Teams and work groups
- Managing change

At any rate, a successful OD effort merely scratches the surface with the above activities. Table 8-5 is an organization development matrix[13] that provides an expansive list and categorization of possible interventions open to organizations. The selection and management of the appropriate programs are major considerations at this stage. However, once begun and carried out correctly, OD never stops. There are three major criteria that, when operational, assure ongoing growth:

1. *Quality control.* This indicates that the interventions and outcomes are of the highest possible quality. Quantity never substitutes for quality in OD. Better the time frame expanded or the "field" narrowed than settle for poor-quality efforts. Dollars, persons, time, and commitment must be invested to ensure the best. The best is often mirrored and maintained; it is a model to continue.

2. *Spontaneous change.* An environment should be established that allows functional though perhaps unplanned changes to occur. Change efforts can "close ranks" unknowingly to concepts not considered by the task force or perceived as acceptable by a line manager. It is important to support and encourage any additive changes made at any level of the organization. A norm to this effect is often initiated.

3. *Ongoing renewal.* Annual forays into new ideas, concepts, assessments, hopes, learning, technologies, and problem identification are helpful in the process of staying fresh. Additionally, investment in the people who are giving is very important; opportunities for them to "fill their wells," to replenish their coffers, and to attend to themselves and their needs must be provided. Such experiences serve to provide invigorating, enthusiastic, and committed human resources who maintain the norm and effort toward continued organizational development.

At this point in an OD program the organization begins to look inward again, sometimes "closing" itself. This is because the investment becomes so intense and heavy that looking beyond the experience can be very draining in light of the major purpose. It is crucial at this time for OD consultants or specialists to assert their neutrality and objectivity. This balancing action and role is imperative for realistic change and assessment to transpire. The OD person also provides needed input to interventions as well as expert help regarding the evaluation process, mechanics, and tools. During this phase the client system learns the basic skill required for the more diffuse evaluation that is the primary focus of Phase V.

Phase V: Ongoing and regular examination of the "total OD design – organizational progress relationship"

Whereas Phase IV is concerned with the evaluation of distinct parts, Phase V is concerned with the wide spectrum: "What is the relationship between our OD program and organization development? Are we achieving our goals? What new focuses might we make? What emerging issues require rethinking or new efforts?" Equally important, the task force team asks "How are we doing?" This process normally occurs every 12 months with quarterly mini-sessions aimed at identifying any major shifts and readjusting. During this phase, the task force assumes primary responsibility for designing its own process and annual off-site assessment events. The OD professional gradually has withdrawn by carefully transferring to the organization the skills necessary to carry on, to maintain, and to grow. It is this quality of OD consultants that most distinguishes them from other consultant groups: the quality of working to reduce the organization's dependence on them by teaching organizational members the concepts and tools to become independent and successful. This does not mean, however, that experts are no longer required; experts in a variety of areas will continue to be tapped, but knowing when and how to incorporate their offerings will be a skill well learned. One kind of expertise will probably be that of a trusted process observer; it is this role (in combination with general resources) that the OD professional can offer on a continuous basis. The time frame from Phase I to the first meeting of Phase V usually consists of between 2 and 3 years. The intimate knowledge of the client system held by the OD consultant must not be sacrificed; rather, it should be rechanneled according to the growth of the organization and its membership. Process observer and general resource are only two of the more common ongoing uses of the successful OD consultant.

Phase VI: Organizational clarification—Who are we now?

Depending on several variables, each organization sets up a regular organizational clarification period and process. Usually, unless there is rapid change, every 4 years is appropriate to "start all over again." The phases are the same; the differences usually have to do with task force membership, with organizational comfort with the process, and with the involvement level and activity of the OD specialist. Also a significant difference between the first OD thrust and those that follow has to do with the nature of the goals. The first thrust tends to concern itself with remedial action taking—that is, solving problems. Succeeding OD programs tend to be preventive and promotive in their orientation, actively focusing on *health* rather than on illness.

OD in retrospect

Whatever the OD approach helps an organization to learn, its ultimate payoff is in whether or not it improves the quality of work life of the organization member and the quality of work of the organization. Organizational development is a scientifically sound approach because it helps people know to what they can realistically aspire and how they can achieve their aspirations.

THE PEOPLE IN OD

The people involved in an OD program include (1) the task force members, (2) the organization's members, and (3) the professional change agent

(OD consultant or specialist). Each has particular roles and responsibilities within an OD program, some of which have been discussed in the previous section. Their common thread in OD is change. Specialists in OD are *professional change agents;* organizational representatives (the task force) are *participant change agents;* and organization members undergo many change experiences. (The organization is called the change or client system.) Organizational development consultants are *not* organizational or industrial psychologists, management consultants, counselors, or social-industrial engineers; they are part of a separate profession whose training focuses heavily on dimensions of change agentry. The task force members are managers, administrators, employees who belong to and who invest in organizational well-being. Determining membership and the criteria for doing so are important activities. Deciding on who is part of the task force and the task force's character has ramifications in such areas as credibility, acceptance, quality—key elements in OD and in achieving success through an OD effort. The hospital president or administrator is a part of this group of internal change agents; most often he or she is a person who wants the hospital to grow and recognizes that it cannot be run like a small organization or like it has been run—in other words, that it must change. At the outset, organization members must be willing to examine changes and newness. Later, they begin to contribute actively to the promotion and design of change in operation, relationships, and self.

Contracting

How do these groups come together? A description of the process occurring between the task force and other organization members is provided in the preceding section. The focus here is primarily on how the OD consultant and the organization come together. This may occur in many ways, from actively seeking one another out to building on an already existing relationship. The key element is the clarification of the nature of the relationship before any other activity occurs. This is usually accomplished through the process of contracting.

> Contracting is a process through which the client and consultant share expectations and reach agreement about the basic structure of their relationship. Decisions made during a contracting period affect the relationship that is to exist over a period of years. It is, therefore, a very significant event in the life of a change effort. For that reason, contracting may take a considerable amount of time; the goal of a contract and/or a contracting process is to help the client to understand what the change activity is about and its implications for organizational, group, and individual functioning. Thus, the client can make a free and informal commitment to the process— a commitment that will help to make the data collection and feedback activity useful and constructive.[22]

Provided below is a listing of some of the typical elements and questions to be answered in the contracting process.

Establishing a basis for commonality

Upon completion of the OD contracting process, the consultant and task force become colleagues in the process. As discussed earlier, Phase I of OD is organizational clarification. However, before this activity many OD consultants and task forces come together through the building of common vocabulary, understandings, and interpersonal skills. The following list describes an appropriate sequence of primary activity modules necessary to accomplish the commonality:

- Self-awareness
- Interpersonal communications
- What is OD and its applications?
- Change processes and theory
- Helping relationships
- Team building
- Leadership styles and skills
- Power and influence
- Conflict, confrontation, collaboration
- Goal setting

Professional change agents: skills, knowledge, values

How are these two groups colleagues? As change agents. Professional OD consultants have extensive training and education in the knowledge, skills,

---

BASIC ELEMENTS OF A CLIENT-CONSULTANT CONTRACT*

1. What are the goals of the relationship or project?
2. Who is the client and who will direct the project?
3. What kinds of data will be collected and (in general terms) how will the data be collected?
4. How will the data be used (include the procedures and resources to be used)?
5. Who will have access to the data and in what form?
6. What are the estimated time periods for the different activities?
7. How will the project be evaluated and by whom?
8. What resources will be provided by the consultant?
9. What resources will be provided by the client?
10. What process will be used to review the relationship?

*From Nadler, D.A.: Feedback and organizational development: using data-based methods, Reading, Mass., © 1977, Addison-Wesley Publishing Co., Table 5.2. Reprinted with permission.

and values of change agentry. The discussion that follows attempts to underscore this preparation. Though the point here is to define for the reader the expertise of the OD consultant, the information presented also defines the new learning that usually occurs for task force (participant) change agents.

Self-awareness: change. Although the OD consultant must be aware of self in many areas, knowing one's self in terms of change is of paramount importance. Professional change agents spend years in looking at their own beliefs and personal attitudes about change as well as resistance issues. Three assessment tools for aiding new change agents in this kind of self-exploration are provided below.

Change agent concerns. Change agents have a variety of concerns that they keep uppermost in their thoughts and considerations. These concerns serve as the backbone for defining their relationships and differing situations in a professional manner. A listing of these concerns and a brief descriptive statement about each are provided on p. 277. After reviewing these, the change agent may periodically ask the questions: "What concern would be most helpful for me to explore personally and to learn about at this point to develop or improve my change agent capabilities? Why?"

Change agent skills. Although the OD consultant has a variety of skills — educating, consulting, helping, training — change agent skills are very important to the OD effort. The list on pp. 278-279 defines skills in seven areas of

Text continued on p. 280.

DO YOU RESIST CHANGE?
A self-assessment form

SOME REASONS I MAY RESIST CHANGE

1. In some instances, an organizational change can make obsolete the knowledge and skills I have acquired.
2. Change can be disrupting. A break in my established routine may force me to think instead of daydream, to take risks rather than remain secure, and to work hard instead of loaf.
3. Because of personality characteristics, attitudes, and values, I may be predisposed to minimize the risks and make changes slowly.
4. Because peer cooperation is required for success in many jobs, I may be unable to withstand work group pressures and support organizational change.
5. When I am affected by change and ignorant concerning its purpose and implications, I am unlikely to support it.
6. Social relationships that develop at work are important. I will probably resist any change that threatens to disrupt my friendships.
7. When frequent and rapid changes are made, I usually experience an unhealthy level of stress.

DO YOU RESIST CHANGE?—cont'd

WHY DO YOU THINK YOU RESIST CHANGE?

List *three* reasons.

1. _____
   _____
   _____

2. _____
   _____
   _____

3. _____
   _____
   _____

BELIEFS ABOUT CHANGE: A personal and group activity

Check whether you believe the following statements are true, sometimes true, or false. In the space provided under each statement, expand on why you responded as you did.

	True	Sometimes true	False
1. People tend to resist change.	___	___	___
2. Only large or momentous changes are worthwhile.	___	___	___
3. Nothing can be changed overnight.	___	___	___
4. Change means improvement.	___	___	___
5. Change brings hardships for some.	___	___	___
6. Change brings reward for the instigators.	___	___	___
7. No change is possible in a bureaucracy.	___	___	___
8. Technological change should be slowed.	___	___	___
9. Change usually comes by change.	___	___	___
10. People can adapt to any change.	___	___	___

This exercise will get you thinking about how you feel about change and your role in instigating and implementing change. You might notice how your approach to planning and implementing strategies is affected by your attitudes toward change.

If you answered "True" to questions 2, 4, 6, and 10, it may indicate a need to be a little more realistic. If you answered "True" to questions 7 and 8, this may indicate a pessimistic attitude that may make it hard for you to work energetically for change. If you answered "True" to questions 1, 3, and 5, it indicates a recognition of the real problems involved in change.

Continued.

DO YOU RESIST CHANGE?—cont'd

SELF-ASSESSMENT: Personal attitudes toward organizational change

1. All organizations—even the most stable ones—are in a continual process of change.

    Agree   Disagree

    1   2   3   4   5   6   7

2. Organizations that change too slowly or that change in the wrong direction decline and eventually die.

    Agree   Disagree

    1   2   3   4   5   6   7

3. Organizations are like biological organisms; they must constantly engage in adaptive behavior to survive and grow.

    Agree   Disagree

    1   2   3   4   5   6   7

4. Organizations *must* adapt to external changes in the law, natural resources, technology, personnel demands, customer preferences, and competitors' actions.

    Agree   Disagree

    1   2   3   4   5   6   7

5. Internal changes, made in response to environmental demands, tend to affect the entire system, often in predictable ways.

    Agree   Disagree

    1   2   3   4   5   6   7

6. A delicate balance must be maintained between demands for continual change and the necessity for organizational stability.

    Agree   Disagree

    1   2   3   4   5   6   7

7. One of the major challenges with which organizations are faced is the creation of an atmosphere in which rapid, meaningful change is possible.

    Agree   Disagree

    1   2   3   4   5   6   7

8. In recent years the rate of change within American society as a whole has accelerated rapidly.

    Agree   Disagree

    1   2   3   4   5   6   7

9. An economic recession or a change in the chief executive officer may send shock waves throughout the organization and demand signficant change at every level.

    Agree   Disagree

    1   2   3   4   5   6   7

CHANGE AGENT CONCERNS

The following areas of concern are common to most relationships between change agent and client organization (small group, department, corporation—any system).

1. **SELF-AWARENESS**

   Aware of one's own personal needs that might be served in the change agent—organization relationship

2. **ENTRY**

   Entering (and reentering) the organization as a change agent
   Able to work out a relationship that has the desired long-run consequences

3. **DIAGNOSIS**

   Examination of the motive of the organization
   Problem definition and assessment of barriers

4. **DATA COLLECTION**

   Agreement between organization and the change agent as to the kinds of data to be gathered and methods for doing so and with whom it will be shared

5. **RELATIONSHIP**

   Working out a constructive mutual acceptance of each other's contribution

6. **RESOURCE IDENTIFICATION AND DEVELOPMENT**

   Determining those areas where the change agent and organization can be resources to the process

7. **DECISION MAKING**

   How decisions will be made and getting them accomplished and acted on

8. **BOUNDARY DEFINITION**

   Agreements as to where the relationship and roles may proceed

9. **ETHICS AND VALUES**

   Establishing and maintaining a set of values that are kept clear to the organization

10. **PLANS AND ALTERNATIVES**

    Able to effect and successfully work out specific action plans that are tangible and accepted

11. **CHANGE STRATEGY**

    Change agent's capacity for change and ability to consider and devise strategies that will help the systems to carry out the change plans

12. **TERMINATIONS**

    Altering the relationship as it progresses and finally terminates without undue strain to the systems involved

13. **EVALUATION**

    Building in feedback mechanisms that can continuously monitor the change experience

CHANGE AGENT SKILLS

SKILL AREA 1

Assessment by the change agent of his or her personal motivations and relationship to the "changee" (change agent here may be an individual, a group, or an organization)

Some skills and understandings needed for this aspect of change:
   a. Understanding one's own motivation in seeing a need for this change and wanting to bring about a change
   b. Understanding and working in terms of a philosophy and ethics of change
   c. Predicting the relation of one possible change to other possible changes, or to those that come later
   d. Determining the possible units of change:
      1. What seems to be needed
      2. What is possible to that person
   e. Determining the size, character, structural makeup of group changes
   f. Determining the barriers, the resistance, the degree of readiness to change
   g. Determining the resources available for overcoming barriers and resistance
   h. Knowing how to determine one's own strategic role in the light of the situation and abilities

SKILL AREA 2

Helping changees become aware of the need for change and for the diagnostic process

Some skills and understandings needed for this aspect of change:
   a. Determining the level of sensitivity the changees have to the need for change
   b. Determining the methods that changees believe should be used in change
   c. Creating awareness of the need for considering change and diagnosis through shock, permissiveness, demonstration, research, guilt, "bandwagon," and so on
   d. Raising the level of aspiration of the changee and making aspirations realistic
   e. Creating a perception of the potentialities for change expectations
   f. Creating expectations to use a stepwise plan and to have patience in its use
   g. Creating perception of possible sources of help in this change
   h. Creating a feeling of responsibility to engage in this change by active participation

NOTE: Each of these steps and the skills categorized under them may be pertinent to changing: The person, his or her relations with others, the relations between several others, a total group, a community, or widely held opinion. Actually, each changee becomes a changer at some point in the normal development of the change process.

SKILL AREA 3

Diagnosis by changer and changee in collaboration concerning the situation, behavior, understanding, feeling, or performance to be modified

Some skills and understandings needed for this aspect of change:
   a. Making catharsis possible and acceptable when indicated as a starting point
   b. Skill in use of diagnostic instruments appropriate to the problem: surveys, maps, score cards, observation, and so on
   c. Diagnosis in terms of causes rather than "goods" or "bads"

d. Skill in helping changees to examine own motivations

e. Examination of the relations of one change to other changes possible in that situation and helping changees understand

f. Clarifying interrelationship or roles between changer and changee

g. Skill in dealing wisely with changee's ideology, myths, traditions, values

SKILL AREA 4

Deciding on the problem; involving others in this decision; planning action, and practicing these plans

Some skills and understandings needed for this aspect of change:

a. Techniques in arriving at a group decision

b. Examining the consequences of certain possible decisions

c. Making a stepwise plan

d. Doing anticipatory practice in the carrying out of a plan

e. Providing for replanning and assessment at later stages

f. Providing administrative organization

g. Eliciting and eliminating alternatives

SKILL AREA 5

Carrying out the plan successfully and productively

Some skills and understandings needed for this aspect of change:

a. Building and maintaining the morale of the changees as they try the change

b. Deciding on the amount of action needed before pausing for an assessment of process and progress being used

c. Understanding the effects of stress on changee's beliefs and behavior

d. Defining objectives in a manner that leads to easy definition of methods

e. Creating a perception of the need for relating methods to the goal in mind

SKILL AREA 6

Evaluation and assessment of changee's progress, methods of working, and human relations

Some skills and understandings needed for this aspect of change:

a. Skill in the diagnosis of causes when group action becomes inefficient through the use of measuring instruments, interviews, interaction awareness panel

b. Skill in use of score cards, rating scales, and the like

SKILL AREA 7

Ensuring continuity, spread, maintenance, and transfer

Some skills and understandings needed for this aspect of change:

a. Creating perception of responsibility for participation in many persons

b. Developing indicated degree of general support for change

c. Developing appreciation by others of work of participants who need support action taking most often required of the change agent. It is of interest to note that these skill areas coincide to a great extent with the phases of OD described earlier in this chapter.

The job of the change agent. A professional has certain position or role characteristics. The outline below defines the *job* of the change agent, focusing especially on the phase of initiating organizational change. Again, there is a direct relationship among role responsibilities, the OD process, and self-awareness. The job of the change agent is to assure the integrity of this relationship with whatever system he or she is working (see opposite page).

Self-inquiry: a developmental process. Organizational development and change agent roles have been characterized as a series of dilemmas. One way to explore these dilemmas is in relation to the phase of the OD effort of the client organization. A three-step tool for exploring common dilemmas encountered by the change agent while moving through the OD process is provided on p. 282. The professional change agent devotes much time to assessment and self-inquiry.

Process consultation

Organizational development specialists are especially skilled in *process consultation*. Process consultation consists of a set of activities that help a client system to perceive, understand, and act on process events that occur within its setting. Process consultation requires that the consultant (1) establish a helping relationship, (2) understand group dynamics and organizational processes, (3) intervene so that organizational processes are improved, and (4) pass process consultation skills on to the client. Process consultation, according to Edgar Schein,[27] rests on seven major underlying assumptions. These assumptions are listed below. It is relevant to note that they are congruent with goals and perspectives of organizational development.

1. Managers often do not know what is wrong and need special help in diagnosing what their problems actually are.
2. Managers do not know what kinds of help consultants can give to them; they need to be helped to know what kind of help they seek.
3. Most managers have a constructive intent to improve things but need help in identifying what and how to improve it.
4. Most organizations can be more effective if they learn to diagnose their own strengths and weaknesses. No organizational form is perfect. Every form of organization will have some weaknesses for which compensational mechanisms need to be found.
5. A consultant could probably not, without exhaustive and time-consuming study, learn enough about the culture of the organization to suggest reliable new courses of action. Therefore, the consultant must work jointly with members of the organization who do know the culture from having lived within it.

6. The client must learn to see the problem independently, to share in the diagnosis, and to be actively involved in generating a remedy. One of the process consultant's roles is to provide new and challenging alternatives for the client to consider. Decision-making about these alternatives must, however, remain in the hands of the client.

7. It is of prime importance that the process consultant be expert in how to diagnose and how to establish an effective helping relationship with clients.

THE JOB OF THE CHANGE AGENT

The following aspects of the job of change agent are important in initiating change in organization:

1. Clarification of the problem
   a. Concepts to analyze problems
   b. Skill in analysis; skill in collecting information
2. Assessing change possibilities
   a. Motivation for change
   b. Readiness to change
   c. Resistance to change
   d. Capacity to change
3. Motivations and resources of the change agent
   a. Feelings about system
   b. Technical resources to help
   c. Ability to commit time and energy
4. Clarification of the ethical bases for initiating change
   a. What are the goals of my change efforts?
   b. What values underlie these goals?
5. Formulating appropriate change objectives
   a. Goals emerge from a realistic diagnosis
   b. Work with inclusive group
   c. Select effective leverage points
6. Ability to take appropriate helping roles
   a. Sensitive to what role is needed
   b. Ability to take it
   c. Skills in performing it
7. Building and maintaining effective relationships
   a. Neutrality—identification with goals
   b. How much dependency
   c. When to push—when to question
8. Adapting to the phase of process
   a. Shifting from diagnosis to action planning
   b. From stimulator of ideas to stimulator of action to supporter of action
9. Acquiring—using repertoire of techniques—skills
   a. Skills in setting up learning situations
   b. Skills in providing feedback
   c. Skills in dealing with resistance

SELF INQUIRY
Dilemmas of my change agent role

As I enter this organizational development effort I face certain dilemmas or confrontations about my role and about the development of a meaningful and accepted helping relationship to the client system. Described briefly here are one or two dilemmas as I sense them now in this early phase of the project.

MY CHANGE AGENT ROLE DILEMMAS, CONFRONTATIONS, DECISION ISSUES

(Later)

CLARIFYING THE CHANGE PROJECT FOR MYSELF

1. Who is my client system?
2. What are my change objectives?
3. How do I perceive and define my role?
4. How is my role perceived and defined by the client system?
5. What steps of progress do I think have been made? Feelings of success?
6. What problems, puzzles encountered?
7. What is my plan for helping at this time? What activity, interventions?
8. Where should I like to end up in this effort? What would be the symptoms of success?

(At the end)

AN OVERVIEW OF THE CHANGE PROJECT

Identification of client system

What was the confronting problem or need for change as defined by me?

What was the level of pain, awareness of the problem, and desire for change in the client system?

How was the helping relationship established? Type of start-up, incentive, entry technique, degree of mutuality of "contact," and so on.

What were the goals of the change project?

What was (or is) my diagnosis of the forces supporting and restraining change in the client system; and supporting or resisting my role as helper?

What were the interventions and the responses; what phases of change and resistance to change have I observed?

What have I done to get feedback to measure the effectiveness of my efforts as well as to provide guidance?

What have I done about termination of the relationship and support for continuity of effort?

What important things have I learned about helping techniques, traps, conceptions of the change agent role?

What observations and comments can I make on the consultation experience?

The consulting relationship

There are a variety of approaches to consulting or helping relationships. Organizational development consultants prefer to work in collaboration with their clients; however, it normally takes time and effort on both the client's and the consultant's part to reach this relationship style. One way of understanding the reason for this has to do with what most people are used to in helping relationships: active prescribing from the expert, passive observing from the client. Consulting relationships for OD by definition cannot operate in this realm. Most OD consultants therefore work from the first with their clients to help them move to higher level interaction styles. A summary of this development is presented in Table 8-6 according to the posture assumed by the client in terms of the kinds of *verbal requests* made, the *consultant's role* given the verbal requests, and the natural consequences of the consultant's activities on the *client's role*. This development recognizes a movement consistent with assumptions about how people mature: *from* passive, relatively conforming reactions *to* interpretive, relatively spontaneous models of self and environment. It is not always possible to function in Phase IV; in fact, the process of reaching this highest level of relating tends to match the progress and development of the organization. By the time the relationship is Phase IV, the formal OD effort is just about over and the consultant is planning with the client for termination of the relationship. It is, however, from this posture of relating that OD consultants enter every organization.

TABLE 8-6
Developmental phases in consulting relationships*

Style of verbal request	Consultant role	Client role
I. "Give us a pill." "Take care of the problem." "Tell us what should be done." "Do it for us."	Active/prescriptive	Passive/observant
II. "Tell me what to do." "I'll do it."	Active in diagnosis/prescriptive	Passive in diagnosis/active in prescription
III. "Isn't this right?" "Shall we do it this way?" "Help me to do it better."	Passive/responsive	Active/prescriptive
IV. "Let me do it myself." "Let's do it together."	Collaborative	Makes decisions on action

*Reproduced by special permission from Ruma, S.J.: Social change—ideas and application: A diagnostic model for organizational change, NTL Institute 4(4):16, 1974.

Role and personal characteristics of the OD consultant

One of the best ways to understand the strength and contribution potential of the OD specialist is to examine several requisite role and personal characteristics. The discussion that follows is based on Michael Beer's outstanding discussion in his book, *Organizational Change and Development: A Systems View.*[2]

Roles. The OD consultant is a *generalist* in organizational and administrative perspective and a *specialist* in the process of organizational diagnosis and intervention (in the change process). Generalist capabilities are as follows:

- Understanding of the management process
- Sufficient knowledge about the purpose and fit of various units (marketing, production) and components (people, products, clients, technology) of the organization
- High-level interpersonal skills
- High-level leadership skills
- Model and change catalyst
- Balanced short-term and long-term orientation
- Broad knowledge of administrative and behavioral sciences

Specialist capabilities are as follows:

- Expert in the process and techniques of organizational diagnosis
- Expert in process consultation
- Expert in intervention theory and method
- Expert in dynamics of planned change

The OD consultant is an integrator by linking the client organization with outside resources appropriate to the circumstances or problem. Also, this integrative function occurs by linking change targets and top management and other groups who are affected by or who affect the change.

Characteristics. The OD consultant must be nonthreatening and *neutral.* She or he must be uninvolved, as a primary party, with conflicts that exist within the organization. The consultant has no preconceived commitment to a particular solution or direction vis-à-vis change. The change agent has no career authority over others or personal aspirations for advancement within the organization.

Examples of the OD consultant's sources of *credibility* are: (1) they have a knowledge base regarding the organization and its functioning; (2) they are not associated with past failures; (3) they are associated with at least some successes; (4) they are seen as possessing the competence to be leaders. Credibility is required to generate influence.

Organizational development consultants maintain *marginal* roles in relation to the organization they serve and the disciplines they rely on for help. Successful interventions require that the change agent maintain an appropriate discrepancy in values and viewpoint with the change target. This is especially necessary when a client organization or subgroup has a narrow or short-range perspective.

- The change agent maintains values that enhance healthy organizations (e.g., openness, confrontation of conflict, inquiry, innovation). Members of the client system, however, may not understand or value these organizational characteristics.
- The consultant also must remain detached to see the organization objectively and to confront those variables or conditions that need changing.
- The OD specialist needs both an organizational and an environmental perspective.

Marginality allows the consultant to see the organization as a complex interdependent system interacting with the environment. These roles and characteristics impact positively on the organizations served by the consultant; they also impact heavily on the consultants themselves. The next subsection discusses this latter impact.

Selflessness and aloneness

One of the most haunting facets of the OD consultant's existence is the constant separateness. The role requires a separateness from self as well as from others. Marginality, neutrality, integration, and generalist-specialist: these are especially difficult role behaviors to maintain.

> Such a role is lonely, and it is difficult to maintain a sense of identity from which develops self-confidence and thrust. Only a very confident and interpersonally competent person can play such a role. Even then, change agents require emotional and professional networks. . . . If the role is carried out effectively, it will require loosening ties with political allies, confronting people in power, and taking neutral or marginal positions with respect to important organizational matters.[2]

Organizational development persons must invest in themselves as well. Often, taking time in this investment leads to another form of aloneness. Joseph Baglio, in his essay "Creative Solitude," expresses his feelings quite poignantly (see p. 286).

Because of the need to "give up self" and to "withhold self" so often in their professional consulting relationships, OD persons have recognized the desire to attend to their linking needs. For that reason, they began in the late 1960s to develop networks of professional colleagues with whom they can share, explore, and refill themselves. They "find ways to associate with others in similar roles through informal and professional networks. In this way, they can be exposed to relevant models, new ideas, and emotional reinforcement from others facing similar role problems."[2] The word and meaning of *net-*

CREATIVE SOLITUDE*

The tapping of one's own senses to determine the nature of experience, to make choices, and to be responsible for oneself is often initiated through solitude and loneliness.—Clark Moustakas

Memory. A long time ago, one of my dear always-have-stuck-by-me-friends asked me to define my concept of creative solitude. Both of us had been through Battle Academia peculiar to our campus and we had come together to share wounds, mobilize, and confront the next myths of collegiality. During those cherished times we usually expressed significant dimensions about ourselves, but now I was struggling to describe my alone times—those solitary s-t-r-e-t-c-h-i-n-g-s at self-growth.

I was having a hard time of it. My friend wanted to understand me, but I got lost in analogies and abstractions. I am not good at describing. I am pretty good at struggling.

Moustakas, in *Individuality and Encounter,* forcefully expresses the long ago essence of my dialogue with myself:

The search within for new perspective may be a painful, terrible struggle or it may be tranquil and silent, but when it involves a genuine relationship to one's self, a direction is realized that represents authentic choice. This means shutting off other noises and sounds, and it often means withdrawal, isolation, and total self-absorption.

One of my special tasks during the past eight months of consulting and human resource development work has been to define my personal dimensions and values. I began a notebook. I was becoming excited about my potential journal entries. I turned cold: I was struggling with my creative solitude issue. Again.

In a sense, consultants are "loners," states Surles with remarkable insight—in our own way—we operate alone. Sometimes we travel alone. We work alone, write alone, speak alone, sell alone. And, he continues, we face success and failure alone.

I work with people in groups, but very often my research, designing, and materials development times are solitary and lonely. Books, pencils, yellow pads. Silent, thoughtful, productive hours. Paradox: this is also an exhilaratingly special time. I write. I sit quietly. Sometimes I look out a window and hope to see a mallard or a snow rabbit. And I talk to me. Literally.

So . . . I have been recording notes in a journal to confirm my organization development consultant role. How do I let my friend know that I am unfinished—still imperfect, and painfully aware of my vulnerability? Solitude and loneliness go with the territory. And I cannot be all explained. I think my friend knew this long ago . . .

Clients. During this last year some very fine persons have viewed me as the expert. I have been probed aggressively: tell me what's wrong with us! Tell me what you want me to do, and I'll do it! A few fragile souls (who did not know me) placed my ideal image on a pedestal. There are no OD idols, gods or oracles. And with courage, they pulled me down.

I have seen the great pain of helplessness and confusion, and one time during training—when I refused to help—when I said I will not have your dependence—I will not take the limited freedom you possess—I was greatly punished. In some naive, but distinctive way, I wanted them to feel some of my creative solitude . . .

Surles adds an important footnote to the consultant's role: though we may "seem to be in the mainstream of things, we are on the outside looking in, like an objective reporter . . . but we are not escapists." And this, too, says something unique about my loneliness—my need to discover. To value. To help.

Perhaps we must pause in time . . . to ask more questions, to know the beauty and terror of a creative solitude, to doubt our work, to examine our growth.

*From Baglio, J.: Creative solitude, SMES Dimensions **1**(1):2, Spring, 1980.

working has been adapted by numerous groups and in many organizations for the same purposes. It is a special way of saying "I want your help," and receiving and giving help. It is this relationship and phenomenon and investment that characterizes the people in OD.

THE IMPACT OF CHANGE

Change is unsettling because it requires people to give up behaviors in which they are skilled and acquire new behaviors in which they lack skill. Change usually means uncertainty and ambiguity; these conditions lead people to search for meaning in the situation and then to react in terms of the meaning they construct. If, on the basis of this meaning, people believe they will be worse off after the change, they will resist the change. If, on the other hand, people believe they will be better off after the change, they will support and involve themselves in the change effort.

Organizational development consultants effect change. The impact of change is an important part of the OD effort. As a result, their research efforts have led them to define several conditions for helping people perceive the positive nature of change. These conditions, previously listed on p. 245, recognize that, for the most part, people must be involved in the process of change.

Change can affect organizations positively or negatively, but change does have an effect. Kurt Lewin's analogy is fitting: he likens the impact of change to the rippling on the water that results from an object being tossed into it; it is a given and always has impact to the water's furthest reaches.

"Change . . . inherent and inevitable . . . an element in every human situation . . . is never easy."[30]

A CONCEPTUAL CONCLUSION

The conceptual conclusion for this chapter is really one that fits the very foundation of this entire book. It is based in part on the comments of J. Clifton Williams in his book, *Human Behavior in Organizations*.[32] The rest is based on the views of the authors.

Organizations can survive and attain their objectives only because their members are willing to adapt to organizational demands.

If an organization
- Behaves or promotes immaturity
- Rewards permissiveness or dependency
- Rewards only a few
- Suppresses self-actualization tendencies

then healthy individuals who cannot adapt to the norms of an immature subculture become extremely frustrated and cannot function harmoniously within the system. They usually leave; sometimes, however, the organization becomes very ill.

Our book (and this chapter) speaks to the reader about efforts that promote corporate and individual maturity, interdependence, broadly based rewards, and opportunities for self-actualization. It speaks to retaining professional staff nurses and supporting healthy organizations.

REFERENCES AND ADDITIONAL READINGS

1. Baglio, J.: Creative solitude, SMES Dimensions **1**(1):2, Spring 1980.
2. Beer, M.: Organizational change and development: a systems view, Santa Monica, Calif., 1981, Goodyear Publishing Co.
3. Bennett, T.R. III: Planning for change, Looking into leadership series, 1978.
4. Bennis, W.G.: Organizational development: its nature, origins, and prospects, Reading, Mass., 1969, Addison-Wesley Publishing Co.
5. Bennis, W.G., and Benne, C., editors: The planning of change, New York, 1969, Holt, Rinehart and Winston.
6. Burke, W.W.: The demise of organizational development, J. Contemp. Bus. **1**(3):57, Summer 1972.
7. Burke, W.W.: The role of training in organizational development, Train. & Develop. J. **26**(9):30-34, Sept. 1972.
8. Fisher, D.W.: A review of organizational development, J. Nurs. Admin. **10**(10):31, Oct. 1980.
9. Gibson, J.L., Ivancevich, J.M., and Donnelly, J.H.: Organizations: behavior, structure, processes, ed. 4, Plano, Texas, 1982, Business Publications, Inc.
10. Golembiewski, R., and Blumbert, A., editors: Sensitivity training and the laboratory approach, Itasca, Ill., 1970, F.E. Peacock Publishers, Inc.
11. Hampton, D.R., and Hardison, N.M.: Contemporary management (instructor's manual), New York, 1981, McGraw-Hill Book Co.
12. Harris, P.R.: Innovating with high achievers in HRD, Train. & Develop. J. **34**(10):45-50, Oct. 1980.
13. Johnston, R.W.: Seven steps to whole organization development, Train. & Develop. J. **33**(1):18, Jan. 1979.
14. Lewin, K.: Resolving social conflicts, New York, 1951, Harper and Bros.
15. Lippitt, G.: Managing change: six ways to turn resistance into acceptance, Super. Mgmt. Mag. **11**(8):21-24, Aug. 1966.
16. Lippitt, G., and Schmidt, W.H.: Crises in a developing organization, Harvard Bus. Rev. **45**(6):102-112, Nov.-Dec. 1967.
17. Margulies, N., and Wallace, J.: Organizational change: techniques and applications, Glenview, Ill., 1973, Scott Foresman & Co.
18. McGill, M.: Organizational development for operating managers, New York, 1977, AMACOM.
19. Mead, M.: The changing world of living, Diseases of the nervous system **28**(7):10-11, July 1967.
20. Miles, M.: Educational innovation: the nature of the problem. In Miles, M., editor: Innovation in education, New York, 1964, Teachers College Press.
21. Minter, R.L.: A system for organizational readiness, Train. & Develop. J. **34**(10):52-55, Oct. 1980.
22. Nadler, D.A.: Feedback and organizational development: using data-based methods, Reading, Mass., 1977, Addison-Wesley Publishing Co.
23. Organizational approaches to planned change. In Reading book: laboratories in human relations training, Washington, D.C., 1960, NTL Institute.

24. Plovnick, M.S., et al.: Rethinking the "what" and "how" of management education for health professionals, J. Appl. Behav. Sci. **14**(3):351, 1978.
25. Reilly, T., and Frohman, M.: Initiating and maintaining planned change in organizations, compiled from behavioral science knowledge on planned change, CRUSK, The University of Michigan, Ann Arbor, 1968.
26. Ruma, S.J.: A diagnostic model for organizational change, Social change—ideas and applications **4**(4):16, 1974.
27. Schein, E.: Process consultation, Reading, Mass., 1969, Addison-Wesley Publishing Co.
28. Sherwood, J.: An introduction to organizational development. In Pfeiffer, W.J., and Jones, J.E., editors: Annual handbook for group facilitators, La Jolla, Calif., 1972.
29. Steele, F.: Physical settings and organizational development, Reading, Mass., 1974, Addison-Wesley Publishing Co.
30. Velthouse, B.A.: Planned change: nurses as change agents, unpublished article, 1978.
31. Wisner, J.N.: Organizational change: how to understand it and deal with it, Training/HRD **48**(4):28-32, May 1979.
32. Williams, J.C.: Human behavior in organizations, Cincinnati, O., 1978, South-Western Publishing Co.
33. Zander, A.: Resistance to change—its analysis and prevention, Advanced Mgmt. **15-16**:9-11, Jan. 1962.

INDEX